ELECTROTHERAPY

CLINICS IN PHYSICAL THERAPY
VOLUME 2

ELECTROTHERAPY

Edited by

Steven L. Wolf, Ph.D., R.P.T.

Associate Professor, Department of Rehabilitation Medicine; Assistant Professor, Departments of Anatomy and Surgery, Division of Physical Therapy, Department of Community Health, Emory University School of Medicine; Coordinator, Biofeedback Research Programs, Emory University Regional Rehabilitation Research and Training Center, Atlanta, Georgia

CHURCHILL LIVINGSTONE

NEW YORK, EDINBURGH, LONDON AND MELBOURNE

1981

Distributed in the United Kingdom by Churchill Livingstone, Robert Stevenson House, 1-3 Baxter's Place, Leith Walk, Edinburgh EH1 3AF and by associated companies, branches and representatives throughout the world.

First published 1981
Printed in U.S.A.

ISBN 0-443-08146-8
7   6   5   4   3   2

Library of Congress Cataloging in Publication Data
Main entry under title:

Electrotherapy.

   (Clinics in physical therapy; v. 2)
   Bibliography: p.
   Includes index.
   Contents: Applications of low- and high-
voltage electrotherapeutic currents / Stuart A.
Binder—Neuromuscular electrical stimulation
in the restoration of purposeful limb movements /
Lucinda L. Baker—Electromyography as a
clarifying tool / Dean P. Currier—[etc.]
   1. Electrotherapeutics—Addresses, essays,
lectures.   2. Electric stimulation—Addresses,
essays, lectures.   I. Wolf, Steven L.
II. Series. [DNLM: 1. Electrotherapy. W1
CL831CN v. 2 / WB 495 E38]
RM871.E43   615.8′2s   [615.8′45]   81-38479
ISBN 0-443-08146-8   AACR2

Contributors

Lucinda L. Baker, M.S., R.P.T.
Senior Physical Therapist, Rancho Los Amigos Rehabilitation Engineering Center, Downey, California

Stuart A. Binder, M.M.Sc., R.P.T.
Instructor, Division of Physical Therapy, Department of Community Health, Emory University School of Medicine; Research Associate, Emory University Regional Research Rehabilitation and Training Center, Atlanta, Georgia

Donna C. Boone, M.S., R.P.T.
Director of Research, Rehabilitation Institute, Glendale Adventist Medical Center, Glendale, California

Dean P. Currier, Ph.D.
Professor, Department of Physical Therapy, University of Kentucky Medical Center, Lexington, Kentucky

John L. Echternach, Ed.D.
Director, Program in Physical Therapy, Old Dominion University, School of Sciences and Health Professions, Norfolk, Virginia

Meryl Roth Gersh, M.M.Sc., R.P.T.
Clinical Education Coordinator for Physical Therapy, St. Luke's Memorial Hospital, Spokane, Washington

L. Don Lehmkuhl, Ph.D.
Associate Professor for Research, Department of Physical Therapy, The Institute for Rehabilitation and Research, Houston, Texas; Assistant Professor, Departments of Physiology and Rehabilitation, Baylor College of Medicine, Houston, Texas

A. Joseph Santiesteban, Ph.D.
Associate Professor and Chairman, University of Washington at LaCrosse, Department of Physical Therapy, LaCrosse, Wisconsin

Preface

For the past quarter of a century, physical therapists have been taught that electrical stimulation can have profound effects upon a variety of physiological processes. Yet, until recently, clinicians have viewed the application of electrical stimuli to enhance function, ameliorate pain, or assess neural integrity with a precarious blend of appreciation and confusion. The appreciation apparently stems from an undefined recognition that precisely controlled applications of electricity can positively compliment the "laying on of hands" to benefit recipients of physical therapeutic interventions. The confusion probably evolves from a poor comprehension of the electrophysiological principles underlying the administration of electrotherapeutic and evaluative modalities and perhaps even a consequential fear of many things electric.

Accompanying these perceptions has been the unquestionable onslaught of higher technological advances which, to a large extent, have had an impact upon contemporary medicoelectrical instrumentation. For example, electrical stimulation to evoke spinal or cortical responses for examining central nervous system pathology or assessing the effectiveness of therapeutic treatment was once thought to lie within the domain of a select group of electrophysiologists. Certainly, evoked spinal or cerebral potentials are today very much within the scope of physical rehabilitation clinicians. Transcutaneous electrical nerve stimulation, once used to assess pain perception preceding or following implants designed to modulate pain perception, is a modality now commonly employed by the physical therapist.

We find ourselves in the unique position of actively participating in the use of modern electrotherapeutic equipment. If the feeling that such instrumentation is too complex to be adequately understood and used persists among physical therapy clinicians, then the opportunity to actively participate in the application of recent technical advances will quickly pass us by. This text was written because its contributors felt a commitment to updating our knowledge base in electrotherapy in light of the limited contemporary resources available on the subject. More significant, however, is the common feeling that the information can be presented with considerable documentation and in a thought-provoking manner. Our intent is not to present "cook-book" approaches to the use of electrotherapeutic devices and procedures, although adequate instruction is provided. Our contention is that the clinician should be given the opportunity to understand and think about the principles underlying electrotherapy.

Much of the content is new and does not appear in other texts and monographs on electrotherapy. This notion is particularly true for the chapters provided by Lucinda Baker and Don Lehmkuhl on functional electrical stimulation and evoked potentials, respectively. While most clinicians are familiar with these two concepts, the discussions contained herein are presented with sufficient clarity and detail to enable the reader to gain rapid comprehension *and* to pursue further practical applications.

Stuart Binder has offered a detailed explanation of basic electrophysiological principles and has updated the existing literature on low- and high-voltage stimulation devices. Of particular value in his contribution is an attempt to offer mechanistic explanations for the physiological action of various electrical stimuli. The rekindled interest among clinicians in iontophoresis is addressed by Donna Boone, who provides a detailed historical perspective on this technique and its multifaceted uses.

Dean Currier and John Echternach are acknowledged within the physical therapy community as two of our most outstanding experts in electromyographic and nerve conduction velocity assessments, respectively. Within this text each blends an explanation of technique with comprehensive overviews of essential physiology. The numerous applications for transcutaneous electrical nerve stimulation that are rapidly gaining acceptance among physical therapists are discussed in considerable detail by two superb proponents of this modality, Meryl Gersh and Joe Santiesteban.

Collectively these contributors provide the most contemporary knowledge available in the area of electrotherapy by combining applications and principles in a cohesive manner. Many components within this text may appear to overlap. For example, electrophysiological events are discussed by several authors. Such presentations are quite intentional for two reasons. First, should the reader choose to use this text as a reference or resource book, sufficient but comprehensive information can be obtained within any one chapter, independent of all others. Second, and more important, should the reader select this text as a comprehensive study guide to electrotherapy, presentation of electrophysiological principles from different perspectives will help to identify and reinforce essential concepts necessary to comprehend all existing and many future advances in electrotherapeutic modalities.

In either case, this text is provided in the hope that more physical therapists will pursue an active participation in the use of electrotherapeutic equipment and the multiple benefits that such instrumentation can yield for the assessment and treatment of rehabilitation patients.

Steven L. Wolf, Ph.D., R.P.T.

Contents

1 | Applications of Low- and High-Voltage Electrotherapeutic Currents

Stuart A. Binder

ELECTROPHYSIOLOGIC PRINCIPLES

Electrical currents passed through a biologic system can produce thermal, physiochemical, and physiologic effects. To understand the mechanism of action whereby electrical currents produce these effects, some of the basic terminology and concepts of electricity are reviewed. Next, the characteristics of high- and low-voltage therapeutic current are outlined. Finally, the relationship of the thermal, physiochemical, and physiologic effects of electrotherapeutics to the specific characteristics of clinically used currents will be discussed.

Electrical current is the flow of electrons through a conducting medium as the result of an electromotive force or potential placed across the ends of the conducting pathway. The *ampere* (A) is the unit of measure of current flow: One ampere of current flow is equal to a rate of flow of electrons of 1 coulomb (C)/s. In electrotherapeutics, we usually deal with milliamperes (mA) or thousandths of amperes. The flow of current produces the desired and unwanted effects of electricity on biologic tissue. Therefore, when we talk about the characteristics of the stimulus being used in electrotherapeutics, we are primarily concerned with the current waveform. The rate of current flow depends on two factors: the electromotive force driving the electrons and the amount of resistance offered by the conductor.

$\mathcal{E} \wedge \mathcal{F} \wedge R - A$ 1

Resistance is the property inherent in any material, which opposes an electrical current. The unit of resistance is the *ohm*. One ohm is equivalent to the resistance offered by a column of mercury 106.3 cm long and 1 mm^2 in cross-sectional area at 0 °C.

The material of the conductor(s), length, cross-sectional area, and temperature all determine the resistance of a pathway. For any given material, the availability of free electrons to conduct a current determines the resistance of the material. The greater the number of free electrons, the lower its resistance. Rubber, a material whose electrons are bound closely to their nuclei, has few free electrons and is thus a poor conductor of electricity. Rubber is an insulator. Metals are examples of good conductors. Increasing the length of a pathway increases that pathway's resistance. Increasing the cross-sectional area of a conductor provides more room for the electrodes to move through, thus decreasing resistance. Increasing the temperature of most materials increases the random movement of electrons, which tends to impede the flow of electrons thus increasing resistance. An exception to this thermal effect is seen in some semiconductors. To minimize resistance: the resistance of each part of the current pathway, particularly the skin and the skin-electrode interface must be minimized; the shortest pathway of electron flow must be used; and the largest electrodes that selectively excite the desired tissue must be used.

The terms *electromotive force (EMF)*, *potential difference,* and *voltage* are often used interchangeably. The EMF is produced by the difference in charge (potential) between two points due to an imbalance in the electron population at the two points. The unit of potential difference is the *volt* (V), defined as that EMF which, when applied to a conductor with a resistance of 1 ohm, produces a current of 1 A.

The relationship of the above three factors—voltage, resistance and current flow—is stated in *Ohm's law:* "The current in an electrical circuit is directly proportional to the voltage and inversely proportional to the resistance."

The formula expressing Ohm's law is:

$$I = V/R$$

where:

I = current flow measured in amperes
V = voltage measured in volts
R = resistance measured in ohms

Current flow can be altered by changing the applied voltage or the resistance of the circuit. For example, suppose that a piece of electrotherapeutic equipment is designed to provide a constant voltage output; that is, the current varies with resistance. What would be the difference in the observed response if a high impedance produced by poor skin preparation or inadequate moistening of canvas-type electrodes was compared to an identical arrangement employing adequate skin and electrode preparation? More voltage would be required to produce an identical muscle response when the high impedance electrodes were used. The higher resistances offered by the dead skin, superficial oils, and air-electrode interface of the poorly prepared electrode would inversely affect the current flow, with less current flowing through the properly prepared electrodes. At any given voltage, less recruitment of motor nerves would be observed.

In addition to greater voltages, increased discomfort would be reported when the poorly prepared electrodes are used. With poor skin preparation, essentially a mosaic pattern of areas of widely varying resistances would be observed. These wide variations in resistance would produce discrete areas of high and low current flow. The areas of low resistance, due to relatively high moisture and low skin resistance, would show an exceptionally high density of current flow. This high current flow may produce chemical as well as electrical excitation of the nociceptive nerve endings resulting in pain. On the other hand, relatively little current will pass through the areas of high resistance producing relatively little excitation of motor or sensory nerves.

The way the component parts of an electrical circuit are connected to each other may be described as being either in *series* or in *parallel*. Figure 1-1 shows a series circuit. For a series circuit the current flow has only one pathway. Thus the current flow through each component is equal and the total resistance is equal to

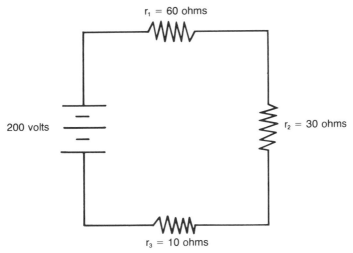

a) the total resistance equals

$$R_t = r_1 + r_2 + r_3$$

$$R_t = 60 + 30 + 10$$

$$R_t = 100 \text{ ohms}$$

b) the current flow through each component equals

$$I = \frac{V}{R_t}$$

$$I = \frac{200 \text{ volts}}{100 \text{ ohms}}$$

$$I = 2 \text{ amperes}$$

c) the voltage drop across each resistor equals

$$v_1 = I\, r_1$$

$$v_1 = 2 \text{ amperes} \times 60 \text{ ohms}$$

$$v_1 = 120 \text{ volts}$$

$$v_2 = I\, r_2$$

$$v_2 = 2 \text{ amperes} \times 30 \text{ ohms}$$

$$v_2 = 60 \text{ volts}$$

$$v_3 = I\, r_3$$

$$v_3 = 2 \text{ amperes} \times 10 \text{ ohms}$$

$$v_3 = 20 \text{ volts}$$

Fig. 1-1. Series circuit. Calculations of (a) total resistance, (b) current flow, and (c) voltage drop across each resistor.

the sum of the individual resistances. Since the current flow is equal through each resistor we note that the voltage drop across each resistor is proportional to its resistances.

For a parallel circuit (Fig. 1-2) the current is provided with alternative pathways to travel. The current flow will take the pathway of least resistance. Thus, the current flow in each of the parallel pathways is inversely proportional to the resistance of the pathway. The voltage drop across each of the pathways is the same while the total resistance is less than any of the individual resistances. Connecting resistances in parallel has the effect of increasing the cross sectional area of the conductor.

Most clinical devices for electrotherapeutics will possess a combination of series and parallel circuits. As an example, if electrodes are placed across an extremity, all of the current will need to pass through the skin immediately under each electrode. This can be considered the series component.

Once the current passes through the skin, various alternative pathways are encountered—fat, blood, muscle, bone, fascia. These are the parallel components. In general, we can correlate the conductivity of biologic tissue to its water content. Muscle and blood are good conductors, fat and bone are poor conductors. Thus, the greatest current flow will be through blood and muscle, and the least through fat and bone.

The characteristics of electrotherapeutic currents include their direction, pulse shape, duration, and amplitude. In direct current (DC), there is a constant flow of electrons in one direction; that is, the polarity of the electrodes are kept

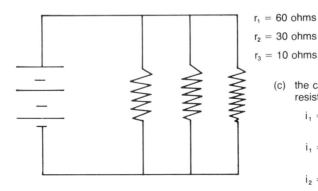

$r_1 = 60$ ohms

$r_2 = 30$ ohms

$r_3 = 10$ ohms

(c) the current flow across each resistor equals

$$i_1 = \frac{V}{r_1}$$

$$i_1 = \frac{200}{60} = 3.33 \text{ amperes}$$

$$i_2 = \frac{V}{r_2}$$

$$i_2 = \frac{200}{30} = 6.67 \text{ amperes}$$

$$i_3 = \frac{V}{r_3}$$

$$i_3 = \frac{200}{10} = 20 \text{ amperes}$$

(note identical voltage drop across each resistor)

(a) the total resistance equals

$$\frac{1}{R_t} = \frac{1}{r_1} + \frac{1}{r_2} + \frac{1}{r_3}$$

$$\frac{1}{R_t} = \frac{1}{60} + \frac{1}{30} + \frac{1}{10}$$

$$\frac{1}{R_t} = \frac{9}{60}$$

$$R_t = 6.67 \text{ ohms}$$

(b) the current flow equals

$$I = \frac{V}{R_t}$$

$$I = \frac{200 \text{ volts}}{6.67 \text{ ohms}}$$

$$I = 30 \text{ amperes}$$

Fig. 1-2. Parallel circuit. Calculations of (*a*) total effective resistance, (*b*) current flow through total circuit, (*c*) current flow through each resistor.

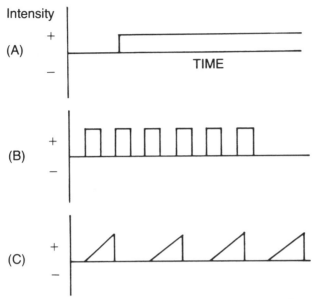

Fig. 1-3.   Direct current. (*A*) continuous, (*B*) interrupted, (*C*) sawtooth waveform. Ordinate is current intensity and abscissa is time for (*A*)–(*C*).

constant (Fig. 1-3). A modification of the DC is pulsed or interrupted DC. In the interrupted DC the direction of current flow never reverses though the magnitude of current flow is not held constant. Figure 1-4 shows examples of alternating currents (AC). In an AC, the magnitude of the flow of electrons constantly changes and the direction of flow reverses periodically. Since there is a constant reversal of the polarity of the electrodes, we never speak of a positive or a negative pole.

The configuration of the pulse shape of both alternating and direct currents can take on many forms. In electrotherapeutics, that characteristic of the pulse shape with which we are most concerned is the rate of rise of the current. We can have a nearly immediate or rapid rise in the application of the current (Figs. 1-3A and B and 1-4B and C), or we can have a slow rise in the current (Figs. 1-3C and 1-4A). The rate of rise of the currents directly effects the current's ability to excite nervous tissue.

The *duration of the current flow* is the period of time the current flows for each individual wave or pulse. This time period can vary from microseconds for interrupted DC or AC to minutes for an uninterrupted DC. The duration of current flow can be manipulated to selectively recruit specific nerve or muscle fibers.

The *amplitude* of the current flow is the magnitude of the current. The *peak current* is the maximum amplitude the current assumes at any point without regard to its duration. The *average current* is the average current flowing between two successive peaks. Thus we can have a waveform with a high peak current though a low average current. An example of such a waveform is the current produced by so-called high voltage generators. The thermal and physiochemical effects of electrotherapeutic currents are primarily a function of the average current, while most physiologic effects are more dependent on peak current.

In addition to the characteristics of individual pulses, most electrotherapeutic currents employ *trains of pulse*. These pulse trains also take on various characteristics. Figure 1-5 shows trains of square waves. Depending upon the interval of time between each pulse, individual muscle contractions or sensations may be realized with each individual pulse. As the interval between pulses is shortened the responses begin to summate. A tetanic contraction or a report of stronger sensation, with the loss of the perception of individual pulses, may be observed if the frequency of stimulation is adequate. The motor or sensory response lasts as long as the train of impulses.

The characteristics of the impulse train can be modified in ways other than the interpulse interval. The current may be *surged* rather than merely interrupted. In a surging current the intensity of each successive pulse in the train gradually increases until the pre-set intensity is reached. A surged current permits a gradual build-up in the strength of contraction as well as intensity of sensation. The duration of each train of impulses and the interval of time between trains can be varied. This on-off cycle time may be used to produce intermittent muscle contractions during an exercise session.

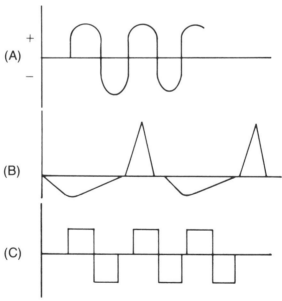

Fig. 1-4.   Alternating currents: (*A*) sine wave, (*B*) original faradic current, (*C*) alternating square wave.

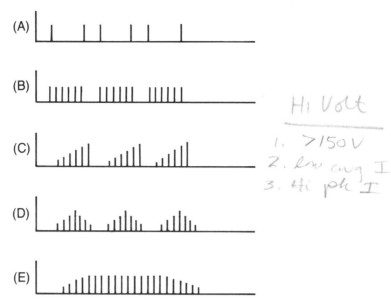

Fig. 1-5. Trains of pulses, (A) individual spikes, (B) interrupted train of pulses, (C) surged build-up, (D) surged build-up and decline, (E) long duration, surged build-up and decline. (Adapted from Scott PM: Clayton's Electrotherapy and Actinotherapy. 7th edn. Baltimore, The Williams and Wilkins Company, 1975.)

CHARACTERISTICS OF HIGH- AND LOW-VOLTAGE THERAPEUTIC CURRENTS

The division between high- and low-voltage currents is more arbitrary than absolute. By convention, *high-voltage generators* produce over 150 V. Similarly, any generator that produces less than 150 V may be considered a *low-voltage generator*. High-voltage generators produce short duration (usually less than 100 μs), high peak (up to 2.0 A), and low-average currents (less than 1.5 mA). The waveform most commonly used is a twin-peaked pulse with 40 to 80 μs spacing between pulses (Fig. 1-6). Trains of pulses, ranging from 1 to 100 pulses/s are usually available with most generators. High-voltage currents may be surged, interrupted or continuous. The high-voltage current is an interrupted DC with the positive or negative polarity given to either electrode.

The particular current characteristics will vary according to the particular application for which the generator has been built. The pulse durations for direct current devices vary from approximately 100 μs to continuous DC. Square or modified square wave pulses with an abrupt rise and fall of the current are most commonly used, though exceptions to the square wave are occasionally used (see Fig. 1-7). Trapezoidal, triangular and saw-tooth waveforms are used to selectively stimulate denervated muscle fibers. Figure 1-8 shows a bidirectional spiked pulse used to prevent the chemical effects of DC with chronic stimulation. This wave is commonly used for cardiac pacemakers.

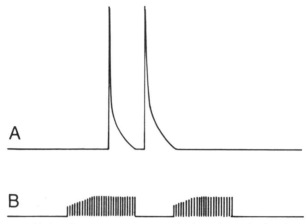

Fig. 1-6. Output of high voltage generator. (*A*) single twin-peaked pulse (*B*) surged output at 80 Hz.

Most of the currents defined as AC possess a rectangular or modified faradic waveform (Figs. 1-4B and C). The sinusoidal wave (Fig. 1-4A) is seldom, if ever, used. The original faradic current (Fig. 1-5B) produced by the faradic coil is now produced by electronic means and consists of a rapid rise and fall of unidirectional (direct) current impulses.[1] The duration of each faradic pulse lasts approximately 1 ms. The rectangular waves may have a duration of .1 to 1000 ms.

The *peak currents* for AC and DC low-voltage devices are relative low compared to the high-voltage devices. The average current for the continuous DC

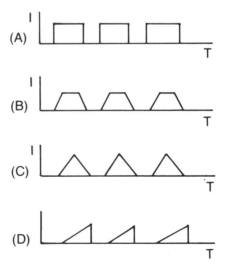

Fig. 1-7. Modified DC pulses. (*A*) Interrupted square. (*B*) Trapezodial. (*C*) Triangular. (*D*) Sawtooth. (Adapted from Scott PM: Clayton's Electrotherapy and Actinotherapy. 7th edn. Baltimore, The Williams and Wilkins Company, 1975.)

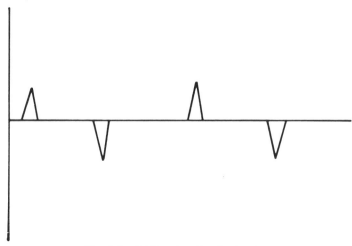

Fig. 1-8. Bidirectional spiked pulse.

may be considerably higher than the average current flow of high-voltage and most low-voltage interrupted generators.

Low-voltage currents, with the exception of constant DC, are often delivered through trains of pulses. Each train may deliver from 2 to 2000 impulses per second and can be surged or merely interrupted. A wide range of the on-off cycle times are presently available.

Biologic Effects of Electrotherapeutic Currents

The passage of an electrical current through biologic tissues produces thermal, physiochemical, and/or physiologic effects. As current passes through biologic tissue, part of the electrical energy is converted to *thermal energy* and heat is liberated. The thermal effects seen are in observance with *Joule's law*. This law states that the amount of heat produced in a conductor is proportional to the square of the intensity of the current, the resistance, and the time for which the current flows. The equation representing the specific relationship is:

$$H = 0.24\ I^2Rt$$

where   H = the heat generated in gram-calories

       I = the current in amperes

       R = the resistance in ohms

       t = time in seconds

HVGS- negligible heat effect due low × I.

For electrotherapeutics, current flow is the average current flow, as previously defined, and time is the duration of the treatment. The principle resistance to the flow of current is that offered by the skin.

High-voltage and the low-voltage interrupted currents used for electrotherapeutics have such low average current flows that negligible thermal effects are produced. The *medical diathermies,* which produce extremely high voltages, do produce significant thermal effects in tissues through which currents flow. For *short-wave diathermy,* depending on the particular electrode placement, the tissues heated may be determined by the relative current flow through them. The skin and subcutaneous fat under the electrodes may be heated due to their high resistance and in-series arrangement (Fig. 1-9). Muscles and blood may be selectively heated due to their high conductivity and resulting high current flow. A high, average current flow is necessary if any appreciable heating is to occur.

The application of a direct current through a solution of electrolytes produces the migration of charged particles towards the oppositely charged pole. When each ion arrives at the oppositely charged pole, specific primary and secondary *chemical reactions* occur. This process is known as *iontophoresis.* The term iontophoresis is also used to describe the penetration of charged particles through the skin using direct electrical current. In addition to the movement of ions, direct currents produce the migration of nondissociated colloid molecules, such as fats and proteins, towards the negative pole. This process is known as cataphoresis.[1] The shifting of the water content of tissues as a result of direct currents, is termed electro-osmosis.

The result of the migration of charged particles produces specific physiochemical reactions.[2-4] The positively charged sodium ions (Na^+), which are in solution within body tissues, migrate towards the negative pole (cathode). At the cathode, each Na^+ gains an electron, forming the uncharged sodium atom. The sodium combines with water to yield the base sodium hydroxide and hydrogen. The increased alkalinity of the cathode produces liquification of protein and the softening of tissues.

At the anode, an acid reaction occurs due to the formation of hydrochloric acid by the neutralization of chlorine ions. The increased acidity brings about a coagulation of protein and a hardening of tissue.

These physiochemical reactions produce specific secondary reactions including a marked antibacterial effect. In 1972 Rowley[5] studied the effect of 0.2 to 140 mA alternating and direct currents on *E. coli* growth in vitro. The results demonstrated a negligible influence for AC on *E. coli* growth with a marked decrease in the growth rate with DC. A 140-mA current showed the greatest effect. This

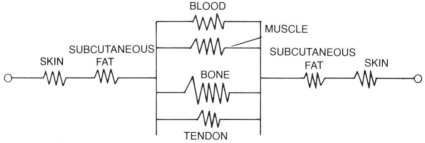

Fig. 1-9. Schematic representation of resistive components of biologic tissue to current flow. Due to the in-series arrangement relatively high current flows through skin and subcutaneous fat. For the in-parallel arrangement relatively high current flows through low resistive components only (muscle and blood).

study also demonstrated that the agent causing the inhibition of bacterial growth was the byproduct of the electrochemical reaction, though not the result of changes in the pH.

Barranco and colleagues[6] showed that *Staphylococcus aureus* growth can be inhibited in vitro in the vicinity of the metal electrodes by the application of .4 to 400 μA of DC. Electrodes made of stainless steel, gold, platinum, and silver were all tested. Both the positive and the negative electrodes were shown to be effective for all metals at 400 μA though toxic effects were seen consistently. Only at the low levels of intensity (.4 to 4 μA) and with the use of positive silver electrodes were the highest levels of inhibition of bacterial growth and negligible toxic effects seen. The authors therefore concluded that positive silver electrodes should be used for in vivo studies.

This suggestion for using the positive pole for its bacteriocidal effects has generally not been followed for most laboratory or clinical studies. Rowley and coworkers,[7] while studying the influence of negative electrical currents on the in vivo growth of *Pseudomonas aeruginosa* on surface wounds of rabbits, found a statistically significant bacteriostatic effect. Probably the best known clinical study concerning the uses of electrotherapy to promote wound healing is that by Wolcott and colleagues.[8] This and other studies[9, 10] initially used the negative pole of the low intensity (0.2 to 1.0 mA) DC generator for its antibacterial effects. The results to date appear encouraging.

While the specific mechanism for the antibacterial effects of electrical currents has not been clearly elucidated, several characteristics of the necessary current have been described. First, a low intensity DC is necessary. High intensity (high average current) would produce unwanted toxic effects.[6] DC is necessary and AC has been shown to be ineffective. Though we know that interrupted DC may produce physiochemical effects with chronic use[11] the specific antibacterial properties of interrupted DC have not been adequately investigated. Therefore, additional information needs to be gathered before antibacterial effects can be attributed to either low- or high-voltage interrupted DC. In summary, at this time only uninterrupted low intensity DC has been shown to have specific antibacterial effects.

In addition to the thermal effects and chemical reactions produced by electrical current, certain *direct somatic and autonomic physiologic responses* are triggered by electrical stimulation. Often physical therapists directly excite motor or sensory nerves to elicit a muscle contraction or reduce pain. Other times, electrotherapeutic currents have been used to increase circulation to promote tissue healing.

To gain a working understanding of the relationship between stimulating characteristics and specific fiber recruitment, the general mechanism for the initiation of the action potential (AP) will first be identified. Next, the relationship between the characteristics of the stimulus, including pulse duration, amplitude, and waveform to the specific fiber population recruited will be discussed. And finally, the mechanism of anodal blocking will be presented.

The general process whereby the nerve AP is initiated is the same for all peripheral nerve fibers; that is, for all nerves, several identical factors related to the characteristics of the stimulus and the nerve determine if the action potential will be initiated. As long as the membrane of an excitable cell (such as nerve or muscle) remains undisturbed, a steady resting potential will be observed. This resting potential, which is approximately −85 mV, serves as the source of stored energy, which allows excitable cells to transmit the action potential. Any stimulus, whether hormonal, chemical, mechanical, thermal, or electrical, serves to depolarize the cell membrane by changing its permeability. If depolarization of the cell membrane is adequate, the cell membrane's threshold is reached and the action potential is initiated. The absolute amount of depolarization necessary to reach threshold is essentially the same for all nerve fibers,[12] though the actual depolarization realized by a single stimulus varies with specific characteristics of each cell. Electrical currents are most often used by researchers and clinicians to artificially stimulate excitable cells because they are the safest and easiest stimulus to regulate.

By the application of an electrical potential across a nerve, a current is passed through the membrane which produces transient depolarization of the resting potential.[12] If the applied voltage is of adequate intensity and duration, sufficient current may flow across the nerve's membrane to initiate an action potential. As with the thermal effects previously noted, the current flow and not the potential serves to initiate the action potential.

Any stimulus that does not permit a muscle or nerve cell to reach threshold is said to be a subthreshold stimulus.[12] The result of a subthreshold stimulus is a local potential. These local potentials are like the properties of electrical cables in that the signal becomes weaker over time and with increased distance traveled. In fact, these local potentials travel only for a short distance along the cell membrane before they completely dissipate. These local potentials are very important for they may actually initiate action potentials.

The time constant (T) of a cell membrane describes the rate of rise and decay of these local potentials following the application and removal of an applied voltage. One time constant is the time taken for a membrane to charge up to approximately 63 percent of the applied voltage or fall to approximately 37 percent of the maximum voltage (Fig. 1-10). The time constant of a membrane is determined by the product of the resistance and capacitance of the membrane. *Capacitance* is the ability of the membrane to separate and store charge. The time constant determines the minimum duration that a voltage must be applied before threshold is reached.

Figure 1-10 is a schematic representation of the rate of charge of nerve and muscle. Actually, the capacitance of muscle is approximately 10 times greater than that of nerve. Therefore, at any applied voltage, the muscle membrane takes longer to charge up to the applied voltage than does nerve. At relatively long duration pulses, both nerve and muscle membrane may be able to be depolarized beyond the level required to reach threshold, but the nerve will always reach threshold first. Therefore, in innervated muscle, electrical stimulation will always occur via the motor nerve. Once the nerve AP is initiated the sequence of events that follow are identical to the events that occur during a normal contraction, save for

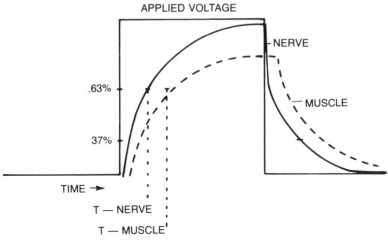

Fig. 1-10. Schematic representation of charging and discharging nerve and muscle cell membranes. Time constants (T) equal the time it takes the membrane to charge up to approximately 63 percent or discharge down to 37 percent of an applied voltage.

the fact that electrical stimulation produces the synchronous firing of all motor units recruited, and the largest motor units are recruited first.

As the duration of the pulse is shortened, higher and higher voltages would be required to reach threshold. There is a minimum duration below which, regardless of the intensity, no action potential can be initiated. From the strength duration curve measurements, we know that the minimum duration necessary to excite muscle would be longer than the minimal duration necessary to excite nerve and that much higher voltages would be necessary to excite both nerve and muscle fibers at the shorter pulse durations. (Fig. 1-11).

As previously noted, the intensity of the applied voltage can be used to selectively recruit various nerve fibers. The amplitude of the current required to excite a peripheral nerve fiber is inversely proportional to the fiber's diameter.[12–14] Large-diameter fibers are recruited with the least applied voltage, while fibers of the smallest diameter require the greatest intensity. The amount of depolarization necessary to reach threshold is essentially the same for all nerve fibers.[12] Due to the characteristics of the membrane and greater cross-sectional area of the fiber, less resistance to current flow is offered by large-diameter fibers. Therefore, for a given applied voltage, a greater amount of current will flow in the larger-diameter fibers (remember Ohm's law, I = V/R). Since current flow actually produces depolarization of the membrane and initiates the action potential, large-diameter nerve fibers are activated at lower intensities than small-diameter nerve fibers.

The threshold for the initiation of an action potential varies with the rate at which the stimulus is applied.[12] This process is known as *accommodation*. The more slowly the stimulus is applied, the greater the depolarization required to initiate the action potential. Thus a stronger stimulus is required. If the membrane

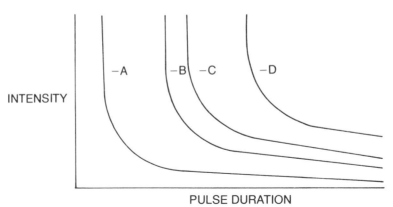

Fig. 1-11. Strength direction curve. Plot of the time versus intensity of current to excite (*A*) large-diameter myelinated motor and sensory nerve fibers (A-alpha). (*B*) small-diameter myelinated sensory nerve fibers (A-delta). (*C*) small-diameter myelinated nerve fibers (C fibers). (*D*) denervated muscle.

potential rises too slowly, the stimulus will be unable to initiate the action potential. The rates of accommodation vary with different cells. Nerve accommodates very quickly and thus an abrupt rise in the stimulus is required. Muscle accommodates much more slowly and stimuli with a more gradual rate of rise may be used.

Based on these physiologic characteristics of excitable cells, certain relationships between stimulus characteristics and specific fiber recruitment can be drawn. If a muscle is partially denervated and we wish to selectively recruit motor nerve fibers only (as is done during some electrodiagnostic testing procedures), we would merely need to use a sufficiently short pulse duration. If, on the other hand, we desire to selectively excite muscle fibers, we could attempt to use one of the slowly rising waveforms previously described.

To selectively activate different populations of nerve fibers, different intensities of stimulation can be used. As can be seen in Figure 1-11, which was taken in part from the work of Li and Bak,[13] the greatest dispersion in the recruitment intensities of nerve fibers occurs at the shortest pulse durations; that is, the short duration of the pulse allows the greatest selectivity in the recruitment of the large-diameter motor fibers. Since pain fibers are of significantly small diameter (Table 1-1), we would expect a minimal amount of discomfort to be felt at the intensities necessary to excite motor nerves with the use of high-voltage devices. Transcutaneous electrical nerve stimulation (TENS) for the treatment of pain also takes advantage of this principle.[15]

In addition to the selective recruitment of different nerve populations, based on fiber diameter, the intensity of the stimulus can also be used to grade the magnitude of the response. We are all aware of the increase in strength of contraction seen with progressively increasing stimulus intensities. This gradual recruitment is in part due to the greater depths to which the current penetrates at higher intensities. The peak current and not the average current determines the depth to which an electrical generator penetrates. Thus, the magnitude of the peak current deter-

TABLE 1-1. Peripheral nerve fiber classifications and function

Type	Class	Diameter (μm)	Conduction Velocity (m/sec)	Function
Afferent				
A	Ia	12–20	72–120	Afferents from primary endings of muscle spindle
	Ib	12–20	72–120	Afferents from Golgi tendon organs
	II	6–12	36–72	Afferents from secondary endings of muscle spindle
	Beta	6–12	36–72	Afferents from touch receptors of skin carrying discriminative touch information
	Delta	1–6	6–36	Afferents from touch (crude), pain and temperature receptors of skin
C	IV	<1	0.5–2	Afferents from pain receptors
Motor				
A	Alpha	12–20	72–120	Efferents to extrafusal skeletal muscle fibers
	Gamma	2–8	12–48	Efferents to intrafusal muscle fibers
B		≈3	3–15	Preganglionic autonomic fibers
C		<1	.5–2	Postganglionic autonomic fibers

(Modified from Willis WD Jr, Grossman RG: Medical Neurobiology., ed. 2, St. Louis, The CV Mosby Co., 1977.)

mines the ability of a generator to recruit deep motor or sensory nerves that do not have a readily accessible superficial motor point.

The frequency of the electrical stimulus also helps to determine the magnitude of the response. At low stimulus frequencies—less than 15 Hz—there is an individual muscle twitch for each pulse. As the frequency of stimulation is increased, a smooth tetanic contraction occurs and the strength of contraction increases. This increasing strength of contraction is due to the summation of mechanical forces within the muscle. As the time interval between successive twitches is reduced, greater overlap of the mechanical process of each twitch is produced. Thus the force of each muscle twitch is summated with the previous twitch and the total force of muscle contraction is subsequently increased. A similar response occurs for the sensory system, with the summation occurring within the central nervous system.

Aside from the application of electrical currents to initiate an action potential in peripheral nerve fibers, textbooks on electrotherapeutics have long identified decreases in nerve excitability under the positive pole of an uninterrupted DC.[2-3] In 1969 Casey and Blick suggested that anodal polarization of nerves may provide a selective, reversible, and easily controlled method to block peripheral nerve fibers from conducting.[16] These investigators found that A type fibers were selectively blocked (alpha, beta, and delta) before the small diameter unmyelinated C type fibers. An orderly blocking of fibers based on diameter within the A grouping was not observed. All fibers slowed before blocking was observed. These findings were confirmed in a more recent article by Whitwam and Kidd.[17] Unfortunately, these authors concluded that the damage produced by the electrical currents rendered this technique unsuitable for clinical use. Hence, at the levels of intensity tolerated by our patients, no real direct sedative effects can be attributed to the anode.

In addition to excitation of peripheral nerves and skeletal muscle, electrical stimulation can cause increases in *peripheral circulation.* Different researchers have attributed these changes to different mechanisms, including the activation of skeletal muscle[18-22] and reflex autonomic responses.[23-26]

The augmentation of peripheral circulation may be mediated chemically through the production of metabolites, and mechanically through the pumping action produced by muscle contraction. In 1948 Wakim and collaborators demonstrated, by stimulating normal, spastic, and flaccid lower extremities, that electrical stimulation producing muscle contraction markedly increased the blood flow in the treated extremity.[22] Extremities that did not contract in response to electrical stimulation showed insignificant increases in blood flow. These findings suggest that muscle contraction, and not simply electrical current, increases blood flow.

Wakim[18] then investigated the effects of muscle stimulation frequency on peripheral circulation. Frequencies of 8 to 32 Hz produced significant increases in blood flow, while frequencies above and below these values showed much smaller increases. At the lowest frequencies too little work was being performed to augment blood flow; at the high frequencies the tetanic muscle contraction interfered with the flow of blood. These findings agree with the work presented by Randall, Imig, and Hines,[19] who also noted precipitous increases in blood flow after stimulation ceased, thus supporting the theory that metabolic and mechanical factors act simultaneously to augment blood flow following electrically induced skeletal muscle contraction.

Electrical stimulation also produces reflex autonomic responses through the direct excitation of afferent neurons.[23-24] Excitation of the dorsal root fibers gives rise to peripheral vasodilation.[25] More recent work has identified early and late sympathetic reflexes in response to the stimulation of group II, III, and IV fibers.[23-24] Dooley and Kasprak[26] demonstrated increases in arterial dilatation with electrical stimulation of the spinal cord or selected nerve roots of patients treated with transcutaneous or implanted electrical stimulators. On the basis of latencies and various other experimental evidence, autonomic responses to electrical stimulation are thought to be mediated at spinal, medullary, and suprapontine levels.[23]

Though direct activation of vasodilator fibers to blood vessels by electrical stimulation is possible, mechanisms for vasodilation appear to have negligible clinical significance. The C-type, sympathetic, postganglionic autonomic fibers supply the smooth muscles of blood vessels. These fibers, which produce vasodilation, are of the same diameter as the smallest afferent neurons from pain receptors. Therefore, a stimulus intensity needed to recruit these postganglionic fibers would also recruit the C as well as the A delta fiber. This intensity would be beyond pain tolerance. Therefore, we may identify two methods by which electrical stimulation may augment circulation: first through the mechanical and chemical effects of an elicited muscle contraction and secondly through excitation of afferent nerve fibers that mediate autonomic activity.

CLINICAL APPLICATIONS OF
ELECTROTHERAPEUTIC CURRENTS

Although the application of electricity has gained popularity many times in the past, only recently has scientific research been undertaken to enable clinicians to draw conclusions regarding the effectiveness of the modalities for specific applications. New suggestions for the use of electrical current grow out of our increasing understanding of the effects of electricity on the body and our ability to produce generators that can meet our desired specifications. Certainly information is needed about the mechanism of action of many electrotherapeutic applications. Each application must be carefully scrutinized and proved effective before it is accepted by the medical community. Most research and clinical reports on the applications of TENS, function electrical stimulation, and iontophoresis have used low-voltage generators. While there are very few clinical or laboratory reports supporting or refuting the use of high-voltage devices, these devices once again appear to be gaining popularity.

One area of research holding great promise involves tissue growth and repair. Numerous clinical and laboratory studies address the growth and repair and soft tissue[18-30] and bone[31-44] following the application of electrical stimulation. Though the specific mechanisms for growth and repair have not been clearly identified, several theories have been proposed and specific characteristics of the relationship of the electrical stimulus to the response have been identified.

Increased tensile strength and rate of skin repair following injury as a result of electrical stimulation have been documented.[8, 9, 27, 28] Bigelow and colleagues[27] studied the effects of low intensity uninterrupted DC (6 to 12 mA) using implanted and percutaneous devices on skin wounds in dogs. The results showed that tensile strengths increased more rapidly for both devices during the first 3 weeks of stimulation, as compared to nonstimulated control wounds. The amount of tissue growth into porous interstices of the neck of the percutaneous device was also measured by identifying the tensile strength between the skin and the percutaneous device. Making the electrode negative increased the tensile strength, while a positive electrode decreased the skin-device tensile strength. Carey and Lepley[28] studied the effects of continuous DC (.2 to .3 mA) applied through subcutaneous stainless steel wires placed longitudinally along an incision in rabbits and found increased tensile strength at the negative pole in the 3-day wounds compared to the positive pole. The tissue about the positive pole showed marked signs of inflammation and necrosis, with thrombi present in many of the small vessels. Apparently tissue growth around the negative pole can be facilitated with implanted or percutaneous devices.

Several clinical studies using transcutaneous stimulation on wounds have also been reported.[8, 9, 29, 30] Wolcott and colleagues[8] and Gault and Gatens[9] studied the effects of low intensity direct current (LIDC) on ischemic skin ulcers. Large numbers of lesions were treated in both studies. Unfortunately, the control group, which consisted of patients who had bilateral similar lesions, was small for both studies. The six control cases in the Gault and Gatens study showed approximately twice the healing rate in the stimulated (30.0 percent) versus unstimulated (14.7 percent) ulcers. Wolcott and colleagues[8] showed 27.0 percent versus 5.0 percent healing per week for their eight bilaterally treated and untreated wounds, respectively. In total, Gault and Gatens[9] treated 100 ulcers and showed 59 percent of the ulcers essentially healed by the end of treatment. Wolcott et al.[8] treated 75 ulcers and showed that 40 percent of the lesions healed completely, and all but one ulcer responded well to treatment. These results are encouraging (though unfortunately not conclusive) when one considers that many of the patients had previously shown either a poor response or gross deterioration to standard methods of treatment.

Assimacopoulous[30] reported the use of negative currents for the treatment of leg ulcers due to chronic venous insufficiency. Good clinical results were reported in all three of these patients for whom conservative methods of treatment had previously proven unsuccessful.

In one of the few published studies of high-voltage stimulation, Thurman and Christian[29] presented a case report in which high-voltage interrupted DC was used to promote wound healing. A 43-year-old female with juvenile onset diabetes mellitus was treated for a purulent, septic abscess on the plantar surface on her left foot. The patient responded favorably to treatment and the leg was saved from amputation.

The mechanism(s) underlying the tissue healing have not been definitively established, but may include: increased peripheral circulation, antibacterial effects, and the direct triggering of tissue growth and repair.

While several studies have shown that negative as well as the positive electrodes may promote tissue healing[8, 9, 27-30] Wheeler and associates accelerated tissue repair with the positive pole.[10] They suggested that the mechanism may be partially mediated through DC feedback signals transmitted from injured tissue to the central nervous system (CNS). The amplitude of the signal would normally decrease as healing progressed. Low intensity direct currents may therefore serve to potentiate or perpetuate the "error signal" so healing is triggered sooner or maintained at a higher rate of repair, compared to normal. This mechanism does not explain the positive results reported for negative surface electrodes.[30] Obviously, additional work needs to be undertaken.

Beginning in the 1960s, many investigators showed that application of small amounts of electric current to bone, stimulated osteogenesis in the region of the negative electrode or cathode.[31-43] Clinical trials using electricity for the treatment of delayed union, nonunion, and congenital pseudoarthrosis began in the early 1970s.[33, 34, 36-42] Constant DC,[36-39, 42] pulsed currents[40, 41] and electromagnetically induced currents have all been used with varying degrees of success. Pulsed currents have generally employed long-duration monophasic and biphasic symmetric[40] and asymmetric[41] waveforms. Invasive[43] (the electrodes, leads, and power supply are all implanted in the extremity treated), semi-invasive[36-42] (only the cathode is inserted into the area of treatment), and noninvasive techniques[33-35] (all equipment is exterior to skin and applied with electromagnetically induced currents only) have all been reported. Current intensities have varied from .5 to 20 mA with continuous DC, and from 30 to 40 mA for the pulsed currents. The peak electromagnetically induced current is reported to be approximately 10 mA.[33]

Recently the work by Brighton, Friedenberg, and Black evaluated the effectiveness of percutaneous, constant direct current on 168 patients with nonunions of traumatic fractures, with an average duration of nonunion of 2.8 years.[38] They showed that 83.7 percent of all patients who were adequately treated healed. Becker and Spadaro, using much lower intensities of direct current to treat 18 cases of nonunions, demonstrated a success rate of 72 percent.[36]

Jorgensen investigated the effectiveness of slow pulsating asymmetric DC on healing time in 24 patients with tibial fractures.[41] A group of 33 patients with tibial fractures served as controls. The treated group demonstrated a 30 percent acceleration in healing, as compared to the control group ($p < .001$). And finally, Bassett and colleagues treated 318 cases of nonunions, delayed unions, and congenital "pseudoarthrosis" with pulsing electromagnetic fields (PEMF) to demonstrate an overall success rate of 80 percent.[34]

From these results one can conclude that all three methods (constant DC, pulsed DC, and PEMF) are clinically effective, but the mechanisms of action have not been clearly elucidated. Different methods have been suggested and include: (1) triggering osteogenic elements by direct currents,[34] (2) promoting the calcification of fibrocartilage by PEMF,[34] and (3) producing local changes in oxygen tensions and pH during the use of invasive techniques.[44] Additional work needs to be done to more clearly identify mechanisms of action and to define optimal treatment parameters.

Another application of electrical stimulation is the prevention of venous stasis and postoperative thromboembolic disease. The cardiopulmonary and musculoskeletal systems both function to help return blood to the heart. The negative intrathoracic pressure during inspiration helps to pull blood back to the heart while the contraction of skeletal muscles pushes blood through the venous system. At the same time, depending on the position of the body, gravity can either assist or resist the venous return.

In 1948 Apperly and Cary demonstrated how the drop in venous return due to a decrease in the pumping action of the skeletal muscle can be reversed by electrically stimulating the muscles of the lower extremities.[21] Findings included: an increase in heart rate and diastolic pressure; decreased pulse pressure, systolic pressure, and circulatory time; pallor; sweating; and distress. Rhythmic electrical stimulation using a sinusoidal current of approximately 20 to 30 mA and at a rate of 18 to 20 contractions per minute helped to return pulse pressure, heart rate, and circulatory times back to normal. Based on their findings, the authors suggested that this technique be used in the treatment of traumatic shock and to prevent postsurgical shock, venous stasis, and thrombosis. The technique may also be used to prevent orthostatic hypotension during standing, following prolonged bedrest or autonomic dysfunction.

Since 1948 many clinical studies have demonstrated the effectiveness of electrical stimulation to combat postsurgical venous stasis and any resulting thromboembolic disease.[20, 45–51] In 1949 Tichy and Zankel,[45] following the refinement of their early work, treated 639 postsurgical patients using sinusoidal electrical current. Two patients (0.3 percent) developed deep venous thrombosis but no cases of pulmonary embolism were noted. The authors commented that 20 or more cases of thrombosis, as well as several cases of pulmonary embolism, would be expected in a sample the size of this study.

Martella, Cincotti, and Springer[46] using a similar approach to treatment, reported no cases of venous thrombosis or pulmonary embolism in a series of 350 postsurgical cases.

In 1964 Doran, Drury, and Sivyer,[47] citing continued occurrences of postsurgical thromboembolic disease, demonstrated striking reductions in venous return from the lower extremities during surgery. These investigators also showed a marked reduction in this intraoperative venous stasis with the use of electrical stimulation to the calf musculature. In 1967 Doran and White[48] reported that the risk of postoperative deep venous thrombosis was reduced by stimulating the calf muscles during surgery. The study was carried out on 200 surgical patients, ranging in age from 22 to 82 years. Each patient served as his own control, as only one leg was stimulated. Comparisons between the stimulated and unstimulated legs revealed statistically significant decreases in the incidence of deep venous thrombosis in the stimulated lower limb (5 stimulated versus 17 unstimulated legs with positive findings). These results were confirmed by Browse and Negus.[50] A similar study was conducted on 110 patients using a ^{125}I-labelled fibrinogen uptake test to document thrombosis formation. The findings of nine cases of thrombosis in the stimulated versus 23 in the unstimulated leg provided statistically and clinically significant evidence that electrical stimulation of the calf muscles during surgery can reduce the incidence of postsurgical deep venous thrombosis.

Anticoagulant therapy, while helping to prevent thromboembolic disease, carries a significant risk in the production of spontaneous hemorrhaging.[49] Of all nonpharmacologic approaches, only elevation, compression stockings, and electrical stimulation have proven to be practical during surgery. Neither compression stockings nor elevation proved to be more effective clinically than electrical stimulation.[49] In fact, Dr. Doran, in a letter published in 1976 in the British Medical Journal, reported that he has gone 10 years in general surgery without serious pulmonary embolism, by using an electronic stimulator.[52] The battery powered electronic stimulator used by Dr. Doran, and reported in the literature,[53] is powered by two 9 V batteries and delivers a 15-ms pulse at a rate of 10 to 30 trains of pulses per minute. Thus, it appears that, though not very popular in the United States, electrical stimulation has been a safe and effective way to help reduce further the incidence of serious thromboembolic disease.

SELECTION OF LOW- AND HIGH-VOLTAGE DEVICES

The selection of a particular device is based on the effectiveness of the waveform it produces and the safety and convenience with which it can be applied. As previously mentioned, few studies supporting or refuting the use of high-voltage generators for specific clinical applications have appeared. Many of the low-voltage electronic generators are compact and lightweight, have been developed for specific applications, and provide the necessary stimulating parameters. The most obvious advantages of the high-voltage generators are their high peak currents and short pulse durations. The high peak current will penetrate deeper and the shorter pulse duration will allow for a more selective recruitment of large-diameter fibers. The high-voltage devices produce no significant chemical or thermal effects.

We can reason that high-voltage devices may prove to be more effective than the conventional low-voltage devices when depth of penetration and selective recruitment of large-diameter fibers are our primary concern. An example of such an application would be for the muscle pumping action produced by electrical stimulation during surgery. Though presently available high-voltage stimulators are larger than low-voltage devices, they may produce better deep pumping. Clinical studies to verify this notion would certainly be interesting. In addition, many of the TENS devices attempt to selectively recruit large-diameter fibers. Based on the characteristics of the waveform, high-voltage devices may be able to more selectively recruit the large-diameter fibers, but do not provide the portability of battery powered low-voltage TENS devices.

Other than portability, the use of low-voltage devices is certainly indicated whenever physiochemical or thermal effects are desired. High-voltage devices could not be used when antibacterial effects are desired. The need for low-voltage devices to promote bone healing or growth has been discussed.

The future of electrotherapeutics is certainly an exciting one. Areas of intense interest do exist. These include research into and the application of stimulation to the brain, as in electroneuroprosthesis, electroconvulsive therapy, and electronarcosis. In addition, cardiac stimulation to save and prolong life is familiar to us all. Finally, the use of electricity to control incontinence and sexual dysfunction appears to have great potential.

SUMMARY

The applications of the therapeutic uses of electricity are growing rapidly. This growth is due both to improvements in instrumentation and scientifically controlled research, which have begun to delineate mechanisms and document results. High-voltage devices presently appear to hold promise for several applications for which low-voltage devices are currently used. Unfortunately, few published studies evaluating the effectiveness of high-voltage devices have appeared in the literature. Such research is necessary if the current popularity of high-voltage devices is to be maintained.

REFERENCES

1. Shriber WJ: A Manual of Electrotherapy, 4th edn. Philadelphia, Lea and Febiger, 1975

2. Shriber WJ: A Manual of Electrotherapy, 4th edn. Philadelphia, Lea and Febiger, 1975, pp. 124–135
3. Watkins AL: A Manual of Electrotherapy, 2nd edn. Philadelphia, Lea and Febiger, 1962
4. Osborne SL, Molmquest HJ: Techniques of Electrotherapy and Its Physical and Physiological Basis. Springfield, Thomas, 1944
5. Rowley BA: Electrical current effects on E. coli growth rates. Proc Soc Exp Biol Med 139:929, 1972
6. Barranco SD, Berger TJ: In vitro effect of weak direct current of Staphylococcus aureus. Clin Ortho 100:250, 1974
7. Rowley BA, McKenna JM, et al: The influence of electrical current on an infecting micro-organism in wounds. Ann NY Acad Sci 238:543, 1974
8. Wolcott LE, Wheeler PC, Hardwicke HM: Accelerated healing of skin ulcers by electrotherapy: preliminary clinical results. South Med J 62:795–801, 1969
9. Gault WR, Gatens PF Jr: Use of low intensity direct current in management of ischemic skin ulcers. Phys Ther 56:265–269, 1976
10. Wheeler PC, Wolcott LE, Morris JL: Neural considerations in the healing of ulcerated tissue by clinical electrotherapeutic application of weak direct current: findings and theory. In: Neuroelectric Research, eds. Reynolds DV, Sjöberg AE. Springfield, Thomas, 1971
11. Von der Mosel HA: Electric signals used for stimulation of muscular tissue. In: Neuroelectric Research, eds. Reynolds DV, Sjöberg AE. Springfield, Thomas, 1971
12. Brinley FJ: Excitation and conduction in nerve fibers. In: Medical Physiology, 14th edn, ed. Mountcastle VB. St. Louis, CV Mosby, 1979
13. Li CL, Bak A: Excitability characteristics of the A- and C- fibers in a peripheral nerve. Exp Neurol 50:67–79, 1976
14. Willis WD, Grossman RG: Medical Neurobiology. St. Louis, CV Mosby, 1977
15. Howson DC: Peripheral nerve excitability. Phys Ther 58:1467–1473, 1978
16. Casey KL, Blick M: Observations on anodal polarization of cutaneous nerve. Brain Res 13:155–167, 1969
17. Whitwam JG, Kidd C: The use of direct current to cause selective block of large fibres in peripheral nerves. Br J Anaesth 47:1123–1133, 1975
18. Wakim KG: Influence of frequency of muscle stimulation on circulation in the stimulated extremity. Arch Phys Med Rehabil 34:291–295, 1953
19. Randall BF, Imig CJ, Hines HM: Effect of electrical stimulation upon blood flow and temperature of skeletal muscle. Am J Phys Med 32:22, 1953
20. Tichy VL: Prevention of venous thrombosis and pulmonary embolism by electrical stimulation of leg muscles. Surgery 26:109–116, 1949
21. Apperly FL, Cary MK: The control of circulatory stasis by the electrical stimulation of large muscle groups. Am J Med Sci 216:403–406, 1948
22. Wakim KG, Terrier JC, Elkins EC, et al: Effects of percutaneous stimulation on the circulation in normal and in paralyzed lower extremities. Am J Physiol 153:183, 1948
23. Sato A, Schmidt RF: Somatosympathetic reflexes: afferent fibers, central pathways, discharge characteristics. Physiol Rev 53:916–947, 1973
24. Whitwam JG, Kidd C, Fussey IV: Responses in sympathetic nerves of the dog evoked by stimulation of somatic nerves. Brain Res 165:219–233, 1979
25. Bayliss W: On the origin from the spinal cord of the vasodilator fibers of the hind limb and the origin of these fibers. J Physiol 26:173–209, 1901
26. Dooley DM, Kasprak M. Modification of blood flow to the extremities by electrical stimulation of the nervous system. South Med J 69:1309–1311, 1976

27. Bigelow JB, Al-Husseini SA, Von Recum AF, et al: Effect of electrical stimulation of canine skin, and percutaneous device—skin interface healing. In: Electrical Properties of Bone Cartilage, eds. Brighton CJ, Black J, Pollack SR. New York, Grune and Stratton, 1979

28. Carey LC, Lepley T Jr: Effect of continuous direct electric current on healing wounds. Surg Forum 13:33, 1962

29. Thurman BF, Christian EL: Response of a serious circulatory lesion to electrical stimulation. Phys Ther 51:1107–1110, 1971

30. Assimacopoulos D: Low intensity negative electric current in the treatment of ulcers of the leg due to chronic venous insufficiency. Am J Surg 15:683–687, 1968

31. Bassett CAL, Pawluk RJ, Becker RO: Effects of electrical currents on bone in vivo. Nature 204:652, 1964

32. Cieszynski T: Studies on the regeneration of ossal tissue. II. Treatment of bone fractures in experimental animals with electric energy. Arch Immunol Ther Exp 11:199, 1963

33. Bassett CAL, Pilla AA, Pawluk RJ: A non-operative salvage of surgically-resistance pseudarthroses and non-unions by pulsing electromagnetic fields. Clin Orthop 124:128–143, 1977

34. Bassett CAL, Mitchell SN, Norton L, et al: Electromagnetic repairs of nonunions. In: Electrical Properties of Bone and Cartilage, eds. Brighton CT, Black J, Pollack SR. New York, Grune and Stratton, 1979

35. Bassett LS, Tzitzikalakis G, Pawluk RJ, et al: Prevention of disuse osteoporosis in the rat by means of pulsing electromagnetic fields. In: Electrical Properties of Bone and Cartilage. New York, Grune and Stratton, 1979

36. Becker RO, Spadaro JA, Marino AA: Clinical experiences with low intensity direct current stimulation of bone growth. Clin Orthop 124:75–83, 1977

37. Becker RO, Spadaro JA: Experience with low-current/silver electrode treatment of nonunion. In: Electrical Properties of Bone and Cartilage, eds. Brighton CJ, Black J, Pollack SR: New York, Grune Stratton, 1979.

38. Brighton CT, Friedenberg ZB, Black J: Evaluation of the use of constant direct current in the treatment of nonunion. In: Electrical Properties of Bone and Cartilage, eds. Brighton CJ, Black J, Pollack SR. New York, Grune and Stratton, pp 519–546, 1979

39. Brighton CT, Friedenberg ZB, Mitchell EI, et al: Treatment of nonunion with constant direct current. Clin Orthop 124:106–123, 1977

40. Herbst E, Von Stazger G: Electrical pulsed current stimulation in five cases of congenital psuedarthrosis of the tibia. In: Electrical Properties of Bone and Cartilage, eds. Brighton CT, Black J, Pollack SR. New York, Grune and Stratton, pp 639–664, 1979

41. Jorgensen TE: Electrical stimulation of human fracture healing by means of a slow pulsating, asymmetrical direct current. Clin Orthop 124:124–127, 1977

42. Lavine LS, Lustrin I, Shamos MH: Treatment of congenital psuedarthrosis of the tibia with direct current. Clin Orthop 124:69–74, 1977

43. Stefan S, Sansen W, Mulier JC: Experimental study on the electrical impedance of bone and the effect of direct current on the healing of fractures. Clin Orthop 120:264–267, 1976

44. Brighton CT: Editorial comment bioelectrical effects on bone and cartilage. Clin Orthop 124:2–4, 1977

45. Tichy VL, Zankel HT: Prevention of venous thrombosis and embolism by electrical stimulation of calf muscles. Arch Phys Med Rehabil 30:711–715, 1949

46. Martella J, Cincotti JJ, Springer WP: Prevention of thromboembolic electrical stimulation of the leg muscles. Arch Phys Med Rehabil 35:24–29, 1954

47. Doran FSA, Drury M, Sivyer A: A simple way to combat the venous stasis which occurs in the lower limbs during surgical operations. Br J Surg 51:486–492, 1964
48. Doran FSA, White HM: A demonstration that the risk of postoperative deep venous thrombosis is reduced by stimulating the calf muscles electrically during the operation. Br J Surg 54:686–689, 1967
49. Doran FSA, White M, Frury M: A clinical trial designed to test the relative value of two simple methods of reducing the risk of venous stasis in the lower limbs during surgical operations, the danger of thrombosis, and a subsequent pulmonary embolus, with a survey of the problem. Br J Surg 57:20–30, 1970
50. Browse NL, Negus D: Prevention of postoperative leg vein thrombosis by electrical muscle stimulation. An evaluation with ^{125}I-labelled fibrinogen. Br Med J 3:615–618, 1970
51. Cotton LT: Prevention of postoperative deep venous thrombosis. Br Med J 2:1193, 1976
52. Doran FSA: Prevention of postoperative deep venous thrombosis. Br Med J 2:1193–1194, 1976
53. Powley JM, Doran FSA: Galvanic stimulation to prevent deep-vein thrombosis. Lancet 1:406–407, 1973

2 | Neuromuscular Electrical Stimulation in the Restoration of Purposeful Limb Movements

Lucinda L. Baker

INTRODUCTION

Electrical stimulation has been used by men of science and medicine for the treatment of patients since ancient times.[1] In 46 AD Scribonius Largus described the use of the torpedo fish to alleviate chronic headache and gout. This treatment continued to be used by both Greek and Roman physicians and throughout the middle ages, although the physicians of that time did find the therapeutic modality to be rather inconvenient. In the mid-1700s, with the construction of the electrostatic generator and the invention of the Leyden jar, a device used to store an electrical charge, electrical stimulation again became a popular treatment modality. From 1744 until the early 1800s many reports were published regarding the use of electrical stimulation in the treatment of hemiplegia, epilepsy, kidney stones, sciatica, gout, rheumatism, and even angina pectoris. Such notable names as Benjamin Franklin and John Wesley were numbered among those who reported remarkable cures with the use of electrical stimulation. In the early 1800s, however, skepticism arose concerning the all encompassing uses of electrical stimulation and the miraculous cures reported.[1]

In the nineteenth century, while advances were being made in the understanding of electrical stimulation and the development of stimulation generators by such notables as Luigi Galvani, Allessandro Volta, Duchenne de Boulogne, and Michael Faraday, little was reported as to its clinical use. Armed with a better understanding of electrophysiology and new devices, such as the battery and the induction coil, clinicians using electrical stimuli once again set off in pursuit of cures for disease. The latter half of the nineteenth century might well be called the golden age of medical electricity.[1] By 1900 most physicians had some sort of electrical stimulation device.[2] Once again, electrical stimulation was touted as the cure-all for various and sundry ailments, including rheumatism, neuralgia, fractures, bruises, cuts, and even insomnia. Electrical stimulation was used to treat diseases of women, to restore manly vigor, and also to exorcise demons.[1]

The popularity of electrical stimulation in treating patients has waxed and waned since the early 1900s. The first article in the journal *P.T. Review* dealing with electrical stimulation appeared in 1922, the second year of its publication.[3] While physical therapists have been primarily involved with the use of electrical stimulation to maintain the bulk of denervated muscle,[4] and, in more recent years, to evaluate the state of denervation in muscle,[5] the use of electrical stimulation with innervated muscle was being explored by the 1950s.[6,7] Since 1961 when Liberson et al. first applied electrical stimulation to help a hemiplegic patient with his gait,[8] electrical stimulation in hemiplegic and, more recently, in patients with a spinal cord injury has become an increasingly active area of clinical research. During the past 20 years electrical stimulation has been used in the treatment of contractures,[9,10] to strengthen atrophied muscle,[9-11] to reeducate innervated but paralyzed muscles,[12,13] to manage spasticity over the short term,[14-16] to facilitate use of an electrical orthosis,[17,18] and to substitute for more conventional bracing. Additionally, electrical stimulation is an effective adjunct to the treatment of pain control in many thousands of patients,[19,20] is used as a phrenic pacing technique to ventilate patients with spinal cord injuries,[21] to assist many paralyzed patients in emptying the bladder,[22] and as an orthotic substitute for the treatment of scoliosis.[23] There are as yet many new horizons to be investigated for the uses of electrical stimulation, but its efficacy as a therapeutic modality has now been firmly established and no longer rests on the extravagant claims of the past.

NEUROMUSCULAR STIMULATION AND CONTRACTURE MANAGEMENT

Electrical stimulation for maintaining or gaining range of motion has been evaluated in both the upper and lower extremities, and with single and multiple joint muscles.[9,10] It was found to decrease knee flexion contractures during a study designed to examine the effects of stimulation on muscle strengthening in atrophied muscle. Munsat et al. described a 33° increase in knee extension range during a 7-week electrical stimulation program of the quadriceps femoris.[9] Despite surgical release of the hamstring tendons, the five semicomatose patients had a mean residual soft tissue tightness of 46° at the knee. An electrical stimulation program was begun immediately postoperatively and after a mean of 6 weeks, the patients' knee flexion contractures had been reduced to an average of 13°. Two of these patients did achieve full knee extension during their treatment programs. During the electrical stimulation program, no range of motion was given, nor were other forms of contracture management attempted.

Based on the results of this study, a similar evaluation of the upper extremity was attempted in hemiplegic patients.[10] Sixteen subjects with wrist and/or finger flexion spasticity were divided into subacute and chronic groups for evaluation. Electrical stimulation was given three times a day in half-hour sessions, and no other form of range of motion or contracture management was used. Electrical stimulation of wrist and finger extensors was accomplished with surface stimulation and carried out either by the patient or by his family after an initial 2-week training period. Evaluation of the subacute patient group showed that range of motion of the wrist, MP, DIP, and PIP joints was maintained. The chronic group of patients, who had some soft tissue tightness of the wrist and finger joints prior to the stimulation program showed a statistically and clinically significant increase in their passive range during and immediately following the 4-week stimulation evaluation (Fig. 2-1). Thus, chronic hemiplegic patients with moderate to

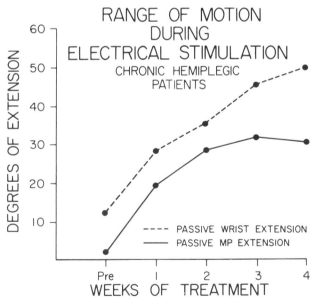

Fig. 2-1. Weekly measurements of passive range of motion of the wrist and MP joints. Average of seven chronic hemiplegic patients treated for 4 weeks with electrical stimulation instead of traditional range of motion techniques. (Adapted from Baker, LL, Yeh C, Wilson D, et al: Electrical stimulation of wrist and fingers for hemiplegic patients. Phys Ther 9:1495–1499, 1979)

severe flexion spasticity, who were unable to maintain range of motion with daily passive ranging, were not only able to maintain but to gain range of motion when electrical stimulation was used as part of their home programs.

From these two studies, it has been shown that passive cyclical electrical stimulation can be a valuable adjunct to present therapy regimens designed to maintain or gain range of motion in patients with moderate to severe spasticity in both the upper and lower extremities.

NEUROMUSCULAR STIMULATION AND MUSCLE STRENGTHENING

There is, at this time, a great deal of controversy concerning the use of electrical stimulation to strengthen muscle. The Russians and Canadians have reported they were able to strengthen the muscles of normal and supernormal athletes by high frequency stimulation,[24] while others have shown no strengthening effect on normal musculature when more moderate stimulation parameters were used.[25] While electrical stimulation in sports medicine remains in question, its use in the treatment of patients with atrophy, either from disuse or from long-term central paralysis, has been evaluated.[9, 11, 26] Munsat et al., in their evaluation of five semicomatose patients, showed a progressive increase in maximal muscle torque with stimulation throughout 2- to 10-week treatment programs.[9] This strengthening effect was largely attributed to an average 37 percent increase in fiber diameter during the stimulation program, as evaluated by pre- and post-program muscle biopsies.[26] In addition to muscle fiber hypertrophy, these and several other authors reported a change in the fiber type composition of the stimulated muscles, with a preponderance of slow-twitch fibers being in evidence after a long-term stimulation program.[27-29] Similar effects of muscle strengthening by prolonged electrical stimulation have been noted by Peckham et al., who also found muscle fiber hypertrophy and muscle fiber composition shifting toward the slow-twitch fiber.[11]

Voluntary muscle torque was found to increase in 10 of the 16 patients evaluated for wrist and finger flexion contracture management by electrical stimulation of the wrist and finger extensors.[10] However, 6 of these 10 patients were among the subacute group of hemiplegic patients, and the increased strength could have been due to spontaneous recovery or to a facilitative effect of the electrical stimulation.

NEUROMUSCULAR STIMULATION AND FACILITATION

Liberson et al.,[8] the first to use electrical stimulation in its modern application, reported that their patients treated with stimulation for foot drop perceived a "carry-over" effect after the stimulation had been turned off. Thus, these patients felt they were able to voluntarily dorsiflex their feet with less effort after a stimulation program and that toe clearance during swing was more natural after stimulation was used. The authors attributed this "carry-over" effect to motor relearning and facilitation of previously paretic muscles. Many other investigators also reported the carry-over phenomenon, with some finding that electrical stimulation was not required after several sessions of treatment.[13, 30–33] While this finding has been primarily reported in hemiplegic patients and patients with head trauma, the phenomenon has also occurred in patients with incomplete spinal cord injury and those with muscle reinnervation following peripheral nerve lesions.[34]

Electrical stimulation to artificially contract a paretic muscle provides a great deal of proprioceptive, kinesthetic and cutaneous sensory input. This heightened sensory input could lead to a new awareness of paretic musculature and assist the patient in learning how to recruit, most effectively, those muscles being stimulated. This notion has been found to be true in electrical stimulation when it is used as an orthotic assist during functional gait activities,[13, 17, 31, 35, 36] and also when used primarily for facilitation. A combination of electrical stimulation with biofeedback has been shown to be particularly effective in facilitating motor control about selected upper and lower etremity joints in hemiplegic patients.[12, 34, 46] While no definitive studies have been done to evaluate the effectivenes of neuromuscular stimulation compared to electromyographic biofeedback, one pilot study indicated that similar results may be achieved by both.[37]

NEUROMUSCULAR STIMULATION AND SPASTICITY MANAGEMENT

Although several reports dealing with the effects of electrical stimulation on spasticity have been reported, the methods used varied extremely.[14–16] Three main uses of electrical stimulation are prominent. The first is moderate frequency stimulation of the antagonist to the spastic muscle.[14, 38] This application has been shown to result in a decrease of antagonistic tone for a varying length of time, reaching up to 30 min after the treatment program has been discontinued. Alternative uses of electrical stimulation are a high frequency stimulation of the spastic muscle[15, 39] and extremely low frequency stimulation of cutaneous areas immediately over the spastic muscle.[16] Investigators examining low frequency stimulation have also reported a carryover effect or a decrease in spasticity. At this time reports are extremely scattered and poorly documented, and further research in this area will be required before a definitive statement about electrical stimulation and its effect on spasticity can be made.

NEUROMUSCULAR STIMULATION AS AN ORTHOSIS

A great deal of work has been done on the use of neuromuscular stimulation as a substitute for an orthosis in both the upper and lower extremity, for both long-term functional and short-term therapeutic uses. Lower extremity orthotic use has ranged from peroneal nerve stimulation as a full-time substitute for an ankle-foot orthosis[8, 31, 35] to stimulation of six muscle groups designed to facilitate early gait training in hemiplegic patients.[17, 40, 41] Stimulation has been used to assist the swing phase of gait in both hemiplegic and spinal cord injury patients, as well as to create stance stability in the hemiplegic patient and upright posturing in the spinal cord injury patient.[42] In addition to various applications to the lower extremity, electrical stimulation has been used to facilitate grasp[43, 44] and release of grasp,[18] to enhance elbow extension[45] and to maintain a subluxed shoulder in proper alignment.[34]

Because the gait patterns of the lower extremity are well defined and stereotypical in nature, electrical stimulation as a gait assist has been greatly refined. Stimulation of the dorsiflexors during the swing phase of gait in hemiplegic patients can assist in alleviating toe drag,[8, 31, 35] while similar stimulation sites in patients with a spinal cord injury often result in flexion not only of the ankle but also of the knee and hip.[34] This procedure can allow adequate clearance for swing and actually create the momentum needed for forward reach and step length in some patients with a spinal cord injury.

Stimulation of the quadriceps and hip extensors during the stance phase of gait can enhance stance stability and allow early ambulation for many hemiplegic patients.[7, 40, 41] In addition, stimulation of the hip abductors during swing can ameliorate the problem of scissoring, while stimulation of greater intensity in stance can provide additional pelvic stability. Stimulation of the gastrocsoleus and hamstring muscles is not used frequently in the United States, however some patients can achieve a better roll-off, and hence knee flexion in swing, by such stimulation.

Multiple channel stimulation is truly a therapeutic activity and cannot be used for long-term, home-based gait assistance. This form of stimulation has been shown, however, to be very effective in facilitating normal gait patterns in the early recovery stage of the hemiplegic patient and in improving gait among some patients with spinal injury.[17, 30] In contrast, single or dual-channel stimulation has been found to be effective long-term therapy, and some patients are able to ambulate while using the electrical orthosis in lieu of other more weighty and inflexible means of bracing.

Because the activity patterns of the upper extremity are so much more complex and diverse than those required for function in the lower extremity, FES has been successful in only certain well-defined applications in the upper extremity. Electrical stimulation to either facilitate grasp or its release in the hemiplegic and spinal cord injury patient has been repeatedly evaluated.[18, 43–47] While several prototype hand orthoses have been developed and successfully applied in clinic settings, independent home use depends on many other varied details of the patient's physical state. Such factors as proximal muscle strength and control as well as sensation in the hand are obvious considerations in evaluating a patient for a hand orthosis.

One area of upper extremity pathology that can be easily improved by an electrical orthosis is shoulder subluxation.[34, 46, 47] Many hemiplegic patients experience subluxation that can be somewhat controlled by the proper use of a sling. However glenohumeral alignment cannot be fully maintained simply by using a sling.[48] Electrical stimulation of appropriate muscles can bring about normal alignment of the shoulder and, with an appropriate training period, patients can tolerate all day use of the electrical shoulder orthosis without muscle fatigue.[46] Thus, shoulder subluxation and its associated problems of pain and swelling can be successfully treated by electrical stimulation, substituting for a traditional sling.

EFFECTS OF STIMULATION PARAMETERS

While several uses of clinical neuromuscular stimulation have been discussed above, the success of these programs depends largely on stimulus parameters. To use electrical stimulation most effectively, the therapist must understand all stimulus parameters and know when and how to adjust them to suit a patient's particular treatment program. Further, an understanding of stimulus parameters will allow the therapist to judge new equipment as it becomes available, and to make an intelligent decision about the best program for his patient. This understanding of stimulus parameters will assure that we do not return to the days when electrical stimulation was an alleged but ineffective cure-all.

Stimulus Frequency   *~ 35 Hz for sm contraction*
↑ > 35Hz lead to fatigue

In using electrical stimulation to achieve the goals described above, a smooth tetanizing contraction of the muscle is usually desired. When a stimulus of one pulse per second is given, there is a definite muscle twitch. As the frequency of the stimulus is increased, the twitching becomes less pronounced and muscle tension increases. As frequency is further increased, the twitching is altogether lost and a smooth muscle contraction is apparent. Depending on the fiber constituents of the muscle being stimulated, this smoothing of the stimulated contraction occurs between 20 and 35 pulses per second (Hz).[49] As the frequency of stimulation is increased above 35 Hz little additional force is gained from the muscle contraction and the existing smooth action is not altered.

The obvious effect of increasing frequency above the smooth tetanizing level is to create muscle fatigue when prolonged stimulation programs are used. The time required to fatigue a muscle by electrical stimulation varies according to the amplitude and frequency of the stimulation, the fiber type composition of the stimulated muscle, and the general state of muscle health. Thus, with all other factors equal, a patient who has not been able to participate in his normal activities or in an active exercise program will demonstrate muscle fatigue during an exercise program with electrical stimulation more quickly then will a normally active subject. There is, therefore, a trade-off between the moderate frequency required to create a smooth tetanized contraction and a low frequency to minimize fatigue. Although this point of balance between moderate and low frequency is

Fatigue Varies
1. Hz health
2. gen health
3. fibers of MM
4. Amplitude

different for every muscle and from one patient to the next, generally the stimulation frequency just above that creating a fused, tetanized contraction will allow optimal long-term stimulation.

During a prolonged stimulation program—lasting several weeks or longer—the muscle's ability to respond to electrical stimulation will improve and less fatigue will be noticed after a 30- to 60-min treatment session. This occurrence may be due to the increased number of slow twitch and oxidative fibers in the muscle, secondary to the electrical stimulation itself. Certainly some muscle groups are capable of responding to nearly continuous stimulation over several hours. This occurs, however, only after several weeks of training the muscle to resist fatigue.[49]

Although the smooth motor response secondary to electrical stimulation is visually similar to a muscle response created by normal physiologic activity, the electrical stimulation is in fact, metabolically expensive and fatiguing. This result from the synchronous firing of motor units when electrical stimulation is used, while normal physiologic activity occurs asynchronously. Thus the motor action achieved by electrical stimulation is due to synchronous firing of some few fibers. The same voluntary muscle contraction may be due to a much larger population of muscle fibers being activated in an asynchronous, low frequency manner.

Pulse Duration

Most stimulators currently available in the United States deliver an electrical current by discrete pulses. This form of stimulation is a contrast to the sine wave generators used from about 1930 to 1960. While not truely galvanic or faradic, the pulse, its amplitude, duration and configuration, determine the type of motor response that will occur. The standard strength-duration curve, defining both rheobase and chronaxie, shows the characteristic pattern of activation of both nerve and muscle (Fig. 2-2). The pulse duration required to activate muscle directly is approximately two orders of magnitude greater than that used to activate the muscle through the intact nerve. Thus, short pulses, regardless of their other characteristics, commonly activate the nerve; therefore, intact peripheral nerves are required to activate a muscle contraction. Pulse durations of less then 1 ms will not be able to activate denervated muscle, regardless of the amplitude applied.

Within the range of 20 μs to 1 ms (0.00002–0.001 s), the duration of the electrical pulse will determine the amplitude required to elicit a nerve and secondary muscle reaction. Thus by maintaining the amplitude at a set level and varying the pulse duration from 500 μs down to 50 μs, a motor contraction of maximal or near maximal strength can be decreased to minimal or no discernible contraction (Fig. 2-3). As can be seen from this second strength-duration curve, as pulse duration becomes shorter, the amplitude required to assure a motor contraction becomes greater. Thus, very short spikes of 20 to 50 μs duration will require a very high voltage output to achieve the same motor response that a stimulation pulse of 300 μs duration can accomplish at much lower amplitudes.

Stimulus pulses of greater than 500 μs have been found, in clinical studies, to be significantly less comfortable than pulses of shorter duration.[34, 46] However,

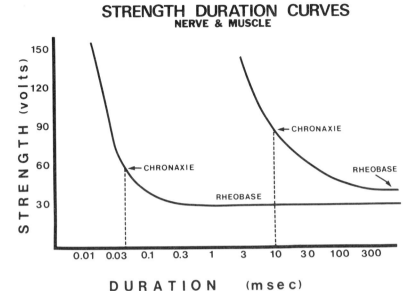

STRENGTH DURATION CURVES
NERVE & MUSCLE

Fig. 2-2. The strength duration curve demonstrates the relationship between pulse duration and amplitude of current needed to minimally excite tissue. Rheobase is that current intensity sufficient to excite both denervated muscle or intact nerve with an infinite pulse duration. Chronaxie is the minimum pulse duration sufficient to activate excitable tissues at twice the amplitude of rheobase. While rheobase values are similar for nerve (left curve) and muscle (right curve), note the difference in chronaxie values for the two types of excitable tissue. (Adapted from Benton LA, Baker LL, Bowman BR, et al: Functional electrical stimulation—A practical clinical guide. Rancho Los Amigos Rehabilitation Engineering Center, Downey, CA., 1980, p. 14.)

pulses of extremely short duration, 50 μs or less, are also found to be uncomfortable, as well as inefficient in activating the nerve. When extremely short pulses or spikes of 50 μs or less are used, the probability that the nerve can be activated while minimizing the amplitude of the stimulus can be enhanced when a second pulse is added. Thus spiking pulses of extremely short duration, when given in pairs, will require less amplitude to activate the desired nerve and muscle response. Stimulus pulses of 200 to 500 μsec have been found to be effective in activating the nerve with moderate energy transmission, while paired pulses of 20 to 50 μsec can also activate the nerve consistently, but require higher amplitudes in order to do so.

One additional characteristic of the stimulation pulse is the pulse-rise time, or the time it takes for the current pulse to reach its maximum amplitude. When the rate at which the current pulse rises is slow, the nerve fiber is capable of accommodation at the membrane level and may fail to spike, despite a seemingly adequate amplitude and pulse duration. Thus, an abrupt rise is likely to activate the nerve more consistently then a slowly rising pulse, as might be seen in low frequency sine wave stimulation.

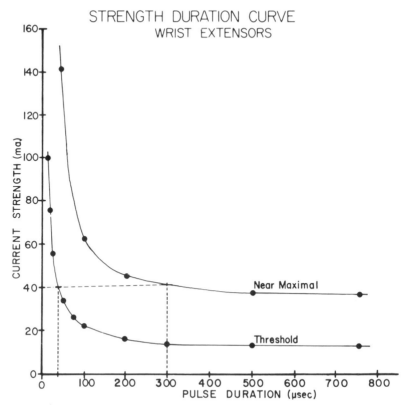

Fig. 2-3. A modified strength duration curve of an intact neuromuscular system, demonstrating amplitude and duration characteristics of a threshold contraction and a nearly maximal contraction. If the amplitude of stimulation is left constant at 40 mA, the strength of the contraction can be varied from minimal to maximal by adjusting the duration of the stimulation pulse from 40 μs to 300 μs. (Adapted from Benton LA, Baker LL, Bowman BR, et al: Functional electrical stimulation—A practical clinical guide. Rancho Los Amigos Rehabilitation Engineering Center, Downey, CA., 1980, p. 31.)

Duty Cycle

The duty cycle is the ratio of the time the electrical stimulation is on as opposed to off. Most stimulation treatment programs use a repetitive ON and OFF cycle to avoid muscle fatigue and prolong the treatment session itself. During the ON time the stimulator delivers a train of individual pulses of prescribed amplitude, duration, and frequency. These trains effect the motor response desired for the particular program. The length of the pulse train, or the ON time, determines how long the response will be maintained. Correspondingly, the length of the OFF time defines the rest and recuperative period for the stimulated nerve and muscle, before the stimulus is reinitiated. The ON-OFF ratio can greatly effect the fatigue of untrained muscle during an electrical stimulation program.

When a patient first begins an electrical stimulation program, a relatively *[handwritten: duty - start by long off work to 1:3 (on/off)]*

long OFF time may be used to assure the ability of the muscle to continue to respond throughout the treatment session. As the muscle becomes trained, the OFF time can be reduced progressively, as ON time is increased to a greater proportion of the stimulation cycle. The limit of a muscle's ability to respond to the stimulation with respect to the ON and OFF times has not yet been established. However, after an extended period of training, some muscle groups can respond to at least a 16-s ON time followed by a 4-s OFF time.[46] The more usual ON-to-OFF ratio is 1 s ON to 3 s OFF. However, 1 s is usually insufficient to create a desired motor response, and the stimulation is frequently given for 4 to 6 s followed by a 12- to 18-s rest period.[49]

Rise Time

A further modification of the pulse train is stimulation with a slow start, or slow rise. The slow rise allows the stimulus amplitude to be increased gradually rather than initiate electrical stimulation abruptly. The advantage is twofold: the patient is not startled by the sudden onset of electrical stimulation and, at the same time, the muscle is gradually stimulated to create a more normal muscle contraction, with more and more fibers being recruited as amplitude of the stimulus or pulse duration is increased. The advantage of the rise time, particularly in spastic patients, is obvious. A quick stretch of spastic muscles may elicit a counter-productive contraction, while a slow rise time allows a slow, prolonged stretch of the spastic muscle and enhances the range of motion and stimulation efficacy.

Obviously, not all stimulation programs can afford the same rise time. Thus, stimulation during gait, required only for a very short period of time, necessitates a virtually instantaneous maximal amplitude. In contrast, stimulation to manage contracture or control spasticity is more effective when a long, slow rise time is used, so that the soft tissue or spastic muscle can stretch slowly.

[handwritten: large fibers easily stimulated]

Amplitude of Stimulation

While we have seen that the motor response can be altered by fixing the amplitude of stimulation and varying the pulse duration, the muscle response can also be altered by fixing the pulse duration and varying the amplitude. The combination of stimulus amplitude and pulse duration determine which nerve fibers will be activated by electrical stimulation.

The large motor fibers, or alpha motor neurons, are the most easily excited by electrical stimulation. However, since stimulation is occurring at the nerve and not directly at the muscle itself, the stimulus also excites the sensory Ia and Ib fibers as well. The large fibers nearest the electrode are activated first and as amplitude is increased, both the large fibers further from the electrode and the smaller axons near the electrode are excited. Activation of the small gamma motor neurons is always accompanied by excitation of the larger fibers and frequently by the small sensory neurons associated with nociception. Thus, electrical stimulation, as used with surface electrodes, activates not only motor fibers and the resultant motor response, but also the sensory fibers and, consequently, the sensory experiences and reflexes mediated by those fibers.

Nerve excitation occurs at the point where the current leaves the nerves. Thus the active electrode is the cathode when a monophasic stimulus is being used. Because the nerve membrane is sensitive to current density, when the cathode or negative electrode is made small relative to the anode or positive electrode, the concentration of ions exiting the nerve under the negative electrode is increased. This results in more nerve fibers immediately under the electrode being activated with a lower amplitude of stimulation.

The motor nerve responds to the amplitude of stimulation with a characteristic S-shaped curve (Fig. 2-4). Thus response and resultant muscle torque are not apparent until a threshold is reached. At threshold, a rapid rise occurs such that

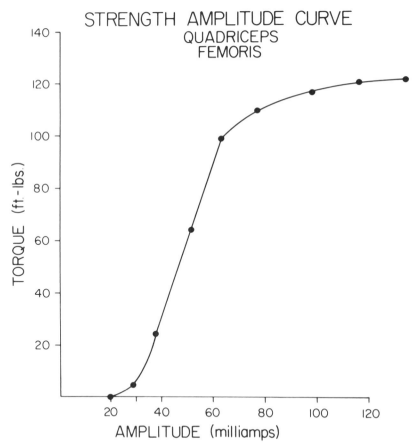

Fig. 2-4. The force output of the quadriceps femoris muscle dependent upon electrical stimulus current amplitude. No torque is produced until a threshold value is reached. Small changes in amplitude above the threshold result in marked increases in torque production, up to a maximal torque output. Further increases in stimulus amplitude fail to produce increased torque, as all available motor units are activated.

with small changes in amplitude a disproportionate number of motor fibers are recruited, until a plateau is reached. At the plateau, all fibers available through excitation by electrical stimulation have been encompassed, and maximum motor output is achieved. The maximum motor contraction by electrical stimulation is greater than can be voluntarily elicited in some normal subjects, due to the synchronous contraction of muscle fibers by electrical stimulation. During voluntary activation, even at maximum levels, some asynchrony may still exist. This greater torque generated by electrical stimulation occurs only for those subjects who have relatively small muscles, covered with little adipose tissue, and then only for some muscle groups and certain electrode configurations. Thus, the force due to electrical stimulation can approach or even exceed the normal range under ideal conditions.

Electrical Stimulus Waveforms

Given today's level of technology, almost any waveform is available from an electrostatic generator. The three most common types are the sine wave, the spike, and the pulsatile currents. As already discussed, the sine wave is not widely used to activate motor fibers in the United States, however, it is used in many European countries. When the sine wave is used, it is usually not at the moderate frequency of 20 to 35 Hz and frequently not with patients, but with normal or supernormal athletes. The spike, by definition, is of extremely short duration and requires high current output to achieve motor contraction. On the other hand, pulsatile stimulation, either of a square wave configuration or some modification thereof, can result in muscle contraction with only moderate voltage output. The standard rectangular pulse shows an abrupt rise in current to a finite amplitude. The amplitude is held for a predetermined time and then abruptly falls back to the baseline.

Pulsatile current can be delivered in a number of configurations, either monophasic or biphasic (Fig. 2-5). A monophasic rectangular wave has the potential disadvantage of causing polarization under the electrodes due to unequal ionic flow, because the current is continually passed in a single direction. Such ionic flow can lead to electrode deterioration and skin irritation, especially when used for prolonged periods. A modification of the monophasic, unidirectional rectangular waveform is an asymmetric biphasic waveform. This wave can take any number of shapes, but allows equal current flow in both directions to minimize skin ionization, while providing a monophasic stimulation effect.

Symmetric biphasic waveforms allow both electrodes to be active during the respective alternating cycles. This effect can be particularly useful when large muscle groups, such as the quadriceps femoris and the gluteus maximus, are to be stimulated.

Evaluations in normal subjects to determine which type of waveform is most comfortable indicate that the majority of the subjects preferred biphasic stimuli,[34, 46] although monophasic stimulation gives a greater degree of specificity. This specificity is particularly important when stimulation of the forearm, hand, or lower leg is desired.

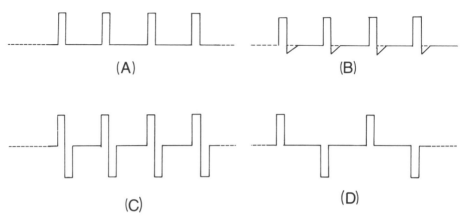

Fig. 2-5. Four of many possible configurations of pulsatile current. A. Monophasic waveform with unidirectional current flow. This results in a single active electrode. Skin irritation due to ion buildup may occur with prolonged stimulation. B. Asymmetric biphasic waveform with current flow in both directions. Because one direction of current flow is of relatively low amplitude and long duration, there is still a single active electrode. Due to ion flow in both directions, skin irritation may be reduced. C. Symmetric biphasic waveform results in activation of excitable tissues under both electrodes. Because ion flow is evenly and immediately reversed, skin irritation is further reduced. D. Alternating symmetric biphasic waveform also creates excitation under both electrodes. When used to moderate frequencies (20–50 Hz) the effect of this waveform is similar to that shown in C. (Adapted from Benton LA, Baker LL, Bowman BR, et al: Functional electrical stimulation—A practical clinical guide. Rancho Los Amigos Rehabilitation Engineering Center, Downey, CA., p. 38.)

Current vs Voltage Sources

An additional factor important in the stimulation waveform is the type of electronic generator supplying the voltage and current. Electrical stimulators may provide constant voltage, constant current, or a waveform combination. Constant voltage stimulators produce the same wave shape and amplitude of voltage regardless of changes in tissue and electrode impedance. This factor can result in unpredictable clinical responses due to changes in impedance during and between treatment sessions when a long duration, multiple application program is being used. A constant-current generator, on the other hand, maintains the same current waveform, regardless of electrode impedance. Consequently the clinical response is more consistent and easier to predict. However, constant current generators must have a safety feature of voltage limitation to avoid possible burns resulting from increased current density if electrode contact with the skin is poorly maintained.

In a study evaluating the sensory effect of current versus voltage-regulated stimuli, there was no clear cut preference for one over the other.[34] In addition, two major centers investigating electrical stimulation use opposite current sources for similar reasons—to insure patient safety. Thus, at this time there are no data to support a preference for one stimulus source over another, although the stimulation response observed during treatment can be better understood if the physical therapist knows the type of stimulator being used.

GENERAL PROGRAMS USING NEUROMUSCULAR STIMULATION

Neuromuscular stimulation can become a major adjunct to many of the treatment programs now being used in physical therapy. This powerful new tool can be used to speed progress in several areas, but it must not be considered a replacement for more traditional treatment. Stimulation is most beneficial when used in combination with standard treatment practices and incorporated into a total regimen of patient care.[49] Many stimulation programs combine the effects of the five major programs that have already been reviewed. Thus, while attempting to increase range of motion, stimulation of an antagonistic muscle may also decrease spasticity and further enhance available range. In addition, during a facilitation program electrical stimulation may provide a strengthening effect of the target muscle. Often, stimulation used as an orthosis can facilitate voluntary control and many times continued use as an orthosis is unnecessary. Thus, combining stimulation with traditional programs may enhance a patient's progress and potentially shorten hospitalization and outpatient treatment.

Range of Motion Programs

Electrical stimulation has been shown to be effective in maintaining range of motion and in correcting soft tissue contractures. Generally a stimulation program aimed at maintaining range-of-motion does not need to be as vigorous as one aimed at increasing range. Thus, a single 30-min program of electrical stimulation may be sufficient to maintain range, even in the presence of spasticity, but a more rigorous 1- to 2-h program may be required to gain range of motion. These sessions may be given in short 15- to 30-min sessions, or in a single 1-h treatment program, depending on the patient's tolerance and fatigue.

The goal of electrical stimulation in maintaining range of motion or in correcting contracture is to allow the joint to move through its full available range. Thus, a fair contraction of the muscle is desired. If the patient is positioned to allow the stimulated joint to complete its arc of motion against gravity, then the joint will be passively returned to its starting position at the end of each stimulation cycle and the patient can be free to engage in other activities. While full range of motion is desired, precaution should be used to assure that the muscle is not creating excessive force at the end of the soft tissue range. This event could result in swelling, inflammation, and pain by 'jamming' the joint into the end range.

Electrical stimulation is particularly effective in such joints as the elbow and knee, both of which are prone to the 'jamming' phenomenon and can easily become painful if ranged too far and too fast. As the joint's passive range increases, the stimulation amplitude can be increased to insure that the stimulated contraction consistently carries the extremity through its maximal excursion.

The amount of stimulation needed for an electrical stimulation program to effectively maintain range of motion or increase range depends on the evenness of the muscle bulk across the involved joint. For example, in stimulating the ankle dorsiflexors to overcome a contracture of the much larger and more powerful plantar flexors, a relatively long stimulation period will be required. In contrast, at the knee joint, where the muscle bulk and leverage of the quadriceps and hamstrings are more evenly matched, shorter stimulation periods are effective.

When using electrical stimulation for range of motion programs, a slow rise time will usually make the patient more comfortable and allow a higher amplitude of stimulation. Thus, a 2-s rise time with a 4-s plateau, followed by a 12-s rest time will usually result in a comfortable program for the patient that can be maintained for 30 to 60 min. If the desired goal is increased range of motion, evaluation should be done within the first 1½ to 2 weeks. By that time some increased range of motion should be noted.[49]

Electrical stimulation in combination with other range of motion techniques is extremely effective. Stimulation can be used during progressive serial casting if either a drop-out cast is used, or windows are placed in the cast over the appropriate motor points. Thus, stimulation can be used isometrically to further enhance the prolonged stretch of the casting. Care should be taken that a cast intended for the combined programs of stimulation and slow stretch fits the patient snugly and has been thoroughly padded to avoid any skin irritation from either the cast or the isometric muscle contraction.

In addition, stimulation can be used quite effectively during more standard stretching programs such as hip flexion stretch. Stimulation of the gluteus maximus during hip flexion stretch may further inhibit the hip flexors and allow a greater gain during the stretching period.

Strengthening Programs

Muscle strengthening programs by electrical stimulation that have been shown to be effective in the past have been extremely vigorous. Successful stimulation programs to strengthen the patient's muscles have involved 4 to 6 h of daily stimulation and have been maintained from 2 to 6 weeks before significant effects were noted.[9] As with the range of motion program, patient cooperation can be minimal with a strengthening program, although stimulation in combination with standard strengthening techniques is extremely valuable. Daily treatment periods need not consist of a single long session, but may involve several shorter periods of stimulation.

Patients with orthopedic problems, including arthritis, and patients who have been immobilized by casts or splinting are typical of those in whom bulk and strength of atrophied muscle may be increased. Other good candidates include patients recovering from upper motor neuron lesions who demonstrate weakness from muscle disuse due to previous paralysis. Patients with peripheral nerve lesions who are experiencing reinnervation, and some incomplete spinal cord injury patients with partial returning innervation are appropriate for a muscle strengthening program as well. Each patient must be evaluated individually, and the extent of reinnervation must be determined to decide if the program will be practical and effective. The number of innervated muscle fibers will determine if increased strength in those fibers will be sufficient to create a clinically significant effect. Because reinnervation can be masked by atrophy and alienation, a short-term trial program may be warranted for patients who show potential for return of muscle function.[49]

Electrical stimulation may be used effectively to assist the patient in actively exercising either against resistance or simply against gravity. Continued stimulation after the active exercise program further exercises the muscles. Care must be taken that the muscle is not overly fatigued by too rigorous a stimulation program. Thus, several 30- to 60-min cyclical stimulation programs in combination with one or two half-hour sessions combining stimulation and traditional strengthening programs may be optimally effective for patients who require strengthening of specific muscle groups.

Facilitation Programs

Unlike the programs for range of motion and strengthening, when electrical stimulation is used to facilitate muscle action, patient cooperation is imperative, since motor facilitation involves supplementing a patient's voluntary response with various motor and sensory stimuli. For these reasons, motor facilitation programs require a higher cognitive awareness than might be acceptable for other stimulation treatments. In addition, motor stimulation sessions tend to be shorter than other programs and ideally are given several times a day. A typical session may last no more than 15 min, and perhaps even less, depending on the patient's attention and participation.

In using electrical stimulation for a facilitation program, the patient must not only participate in his program but must also be able to visualize the activity desired, so that positioning becomes critical for a facilitation program. When electrical stimulation can be combined with more than just visual feedback, the facilitation may occur at a more rapid rate. Thus, electrical stimulation and EMG biofeedback may be used in combination to enhance a patient's own voluntary effort. Cyclical stimulation may not be the most preferred type of stimulation for facilitation. A triggered stimulus can be used to augment a patient's own voluntary effort once he has reached his peak ability. For example, electrical stimulation could be triggered by the physical therapist after the patient has reached his maximum voluntary range of motion at a paretic joint. The stimulation would then augment the patient's own active effort, completing the range for him. After the stimulation cycle, a suitable rest period is required before the patient again attempts to repeat his effort.

Facilitation programs using electrical stimulation are useful not only for the neurologically involved patient but also for orthopedic patients. These patients frequently lack neural deficits but may require assistance in muscle retraining after a period of disuse. Also, neuromuscular stimulation facilitation programs can be used for patients with partially innervated spinal cord injury or peripheral nerve lesions, who have returning innervation but who require concentrated training to optimize their motor control. In addition, electrical stimulation can also be used as a form of sensory facilitation for those neurologic patients who have dense sensory loss. The proprioceptive, kinesthetic, and cutaneous input achieved by electrical stimulation can be remarkably effective in increasing awareness of a limb or a whole side, as required by many hemiplegic patients.[49]

Spasticity Management

While electrical stimulation has been shown to have only a transient effect on spasticity, it can still be used effectively as a precursor to functional training, facilitation, or strengthening programs. As an example, the patient who has spastic hamstrings and is unable to adequately participate in gait training may benefit from a period of quadriceps stimulation immediately before the training session begins. Many times the reduction of tone in an antagonistic spastic muscle can unmask motor control that can be further potentiated and facilitated. Stimulation after temporary nerve block has been shown to be effective in retraining motor control so that the spastic muscle is more normally balanced, allowing increased function, even after the effects of the temporary block have worn off.

In developing a stimulation program for spasticity management, the rise time and ON time must be carefully adjusted. A very slow rise time may be required to allow a slow stretch of the spastic antagonist and to avoid an undesirable withdrawal reflex. With a slow rise time, a prolonged On time may be required to achieve full joint range of motion. Depending on the patient's level of training a long OFF time may also be required to avoid fatigue during the treatment program. Electrical stimulation to manage spasticity cannot stand alone, since the effect does not appear to be long-lasting. Thus stimulation is ideally used to control spasticity, primarily in combination with other treatment programs designed to strengthen and facilitate the underlying motor control.[49]

Orthotic Uses

Two major areas exist for orthotic substitution at this time. The first of these is stimulation of the dorsiflexors during gait to facilitate toe clearance during swing phase, and heel contact. The most appropriate patients for this type of stimulation are those who have adequate calf strength to allow controlled tibial advancement but who lack in anterior compartment muscle control. The electrical orthosis is not adequate to substitute for an ankle/foot orthosis if the calf is inadequate to maintain stability during stance. Several devices currently available are triggered by a footswitch in the patient's shoe. As the patient rolls forward on the toe of his shoe, the heel switch is unloaded, resulting in a signal to the electrical stimulator worn on the belt. The stimulation is triggered and maintained throughout the swing phase of gait until the patient's heel touches the floor, closing the heel switch and thus disengaging the stimulator. This system is very effective both in training the dorsiflexors to spontaneously contract during the appropriate phases of gait, and also as a permanent orthosis for patients who fail to show muscle reeducation. In some patients with spinal injury, the dorsiflexion is compounded by hip and knee flexion, resulting from the activation of spinal level reflexes. These reflexes then allow the patient, who may be dominated by extensor reflexes, to gain sufficient flexion to allow an energy efficient gait.

The second area of orthosis substitution is at the shoulder. Cyclical electrical stimulation to maintain shoulder alignment in the presence of subluxation has been found to be quite effective. Again, stimulation can be used as a training device or as a semipermanent orthosis for patients who fail to show maintained reduction. Stimulation of the supraspinatus and posterior deltoid has been effective in attaining realignment of the shoulder and, with appropriate training sessions, patients can learn to tolerate the stimulation without fatigue for as long as 6 to 8 h. The stimulation cycle of ON and OFF times can be modified over a number of weeks such that the patient's shoulder is maintained in proper alignment for virtually the whole cycle without fatiguing the shoulder muscles.

Electrical stimulation can be used for an orthotic assist in a number of other ways, primarily for training within the clinic setting. Thus, stimulation of the quadriceps, triggered during terminal swing and maintained throughout stance, can assist the hemiplegic patient with stance stability and allow ambulation training earlier in the rehabilitation program. The stimulation has the advantage over a knee cage or knee/ankle/foot orthosis in that it allows more normal knee flexion during swing, as well as proper timing of the muscle contraction. Many reports have stated that electrical stimulation has allowed not only early ambulation but also rapid training of normal muscle sequencing. Patients have been able to progress to more standard treatment programs rapidly, using electrical stimulation in the early phases of their rehabilitation.[34, 46, 47]

Similar to knee extension, hip extension can be used to enhance stance stability in upright posturing during gait and balancing activities, not only for hemiplegic patients but also for patients with spinal cord injury undergoing gait training. This type of stimulation has occasionally been used as a form of semipermanent orthosis. However, equipment reliability must be 100 percent for patient safety if ambulation, or even standing, is to take place independently, without therapist supervision. At this time, patients who have not benefitted from a prolonged treatment program with electrical stimulation for stance stability have proved to be severely involved and are at extremely high risk for a second incidence of stroke. These patients are poor candidates for permanent orthosis. This type of orthotic substitution is used primarily as a training device in the treatment area, controlled and coordinated by the physical therapist.

Other areas of potential orthoses lie in the upper extremity, for both hand opening and prehension, and for elbow control. While therapist-controlled electrical stimulation has been shown to be an effective training technique for both prehension and hand opening within the treatment setting,[43, 46, 47] sufficient equipment sophistication has not yet been achieved for wide scale use on a home basis. However, therapist-triggered stimulation during table top activities has been shown to be extremely effective in training patients to use their voluntary prehension and release. A significant learning and carry-over effect has been documented.[47] Thus electrical orthosis has been useful both in the clinic as a training device and for patients who fail to show training with the in-house device but would use stimulation for specific purposes in either gait or other routine daily activities.

CONTRAINDICATIONS

Absolute contraindications to electrical stimulation are few, and are generally predicted by good clinical practice. The major contraindication to electrical stimulation is cardiac disability. Patients with demand pacemakers should not be placed on an electrical stimulation program. Patients who have any prior history of cardiac dysrhythmia should be monitored electrocardiographically during their initial stimulation sessions. If there is any evidence of cardiac irregularity, stimulation should be discontinued immediately and a physician consulted. Electrical stimulation over the carotid sinuses should also be avoided to prevent any sudden change in blood pressure.

Factors that may potentially interfere with an electrical stimulation program include obesity and diabetes. In obesity, a heavy layer of fat may effectively insulate the target nerve from the surface electrode. The result could be an extremely high threshold to stimulation, requiring a high intensity to achieve the desired effect. Because the surface of the skin and its associated sensory receptors would be subjected to the high amplitude stimulation, the patient may not tolerate sufficient stimulation to achieve the desired effect. Although gradual increases in the level of stimulus amplitude can frequently alleviate a patient's initial fearful response to the sensation that accompanies stimulation, in the case of an obese patient the sensory intolerance may not be overcome. In some patients who tolerate the sensation of electrical stimulation but who are very obese, the stimulator may be unable to put out sufficient power to achieve the desired muscle contraction. In these cases, electrical stimulation, except as a means of increasing sensory awareness, may be unsuccessful.

In the case of the diabetic or other patients who have peripheral neuropathies or partial denervation of a muscle, electrical stimulation may not be able to achieve the desired muscle response. Because surface stimulation can only stimulate those nerves closest to the electrode, not all nerve fibers of a muscle may be activated by the stimulation. Thus, if the most peripheral fibers of a nerve are denervated, the effect of electrical stimulation will be reduced. In some diabetics and patients with peripheral neuropathies, the stimulated contractions fall short of what the patient is able to do on his own, due to diffuse denervation throughout the muscle. Again, unless the desired effect of electrical stimulation is increased sensory awareness, the efficacy of stimulation in treating this type of patient is suspect.

Although the technology of surface electrodes and the gel and tape used to affix the electrodes is constantly advancing, some patients will develop skin irritations. Although skin reactions, when watched for carefully, are not a major problem, they can become a considerable hindrance to electrical stimulation programs if ignored. This is particularly true in the patient with spinal injury or other patients with poor sensation.

The final potentially interfering factor in the use of electrical stimulation is patient acceptance. Because electrical stimulation is a new sensory experience to the majority of people, the initial reaction is frequently one of rejection, particularly if the therapist overenthusiastically increases the amplitude to achieve the desired motor response within one or two sessions. In most cases patients will accept the new sensation of electrical stimulation but require a "warm-up" period. The patient should always be in control of the amplitude of his treatment program and a therapist should not attempt to push the amplitude higher than the patient's sensory tolerance allows. By giving the patient several sessions to become accustomed to the sensation that accompanies stimulation, the therapist can gradually increase the amplitude to ultimately achieve the desired response. In most cases 3 to 4 days of cyclical stimulation is sufficient to familiarize the patient with the stimulation experience and achieve the desired motor response.

The attitude of the therapist, however, is critical in determining how well the patient will accept stimulation. If the therapist is afraid of, or harbors negative attitudes about stimulation, the probability that the patient will accept the stimulation program is greatly reduced. If, however, the physical therapist approaches electrical stimulation in a positive manner, allows the patient to adjust to the sensations of stimulation, and only gradually increases the amplitude, nearly all subjects will tolerate sufficient stimulation to allow an effective electrical stimulation program.

CONCLUSION

Electrical stimulation, a treatment modality known since ancient times, has now become a clinical tool to be used by physical therapists in programs that have been documented through clinical research. As greater technology expands our use of electrical stimulation, new programs based on further clinical evaluations will be developed. Although electrical stimulation is not the panacea it was once thought to be, it does have a valid and valuable place in the physical therapy clinic. Further research and development will continue to expand its use in our treatment repertoire.

REFERENCES

1. McNeal DR: 2000 years of electrical stimulation. In: Functional Electrical Stimulation: Applications in Neural Prostheses. eds. FT Hambrecht, JB Reswick. New York, Marcel Dekker, 1977, pp 3–35
2. Reswick JB: A brief history of functional electrical stimulation. In: Neural Organization and its Relevance to Prosthetics. eds. WS Fields, LA Leavitt. New York, Intercontinental Medical Book Corp., 1973, pp 3–13
3. Gary CE: Interpolar action of the galvanic current, Part I. Phys Ther Rev 2(2):5–7, Part II. Phys Ther Rev 2(3):7–11, 1922

4. Osborne SL, Gradius FS: Electrical stimulation of denervated muscle. Physiother Rev 22:291–295, 1942
5. Ayres WL, Paul WD: Chronaxy changes in rheumatoid arthritis: a study of hand muscles. Phys Ther 47:22–25, 1967
6. Hartmann AC, Bowman HD: Influence of electrical stimulation of muscles on the development of fatigue in man. Phys Ther Rev 30:363–370, 1950
7. Weinstein MV, Gordon A: Use of faradism in the rehabilitation of hemiplegics. Phys Ther Rev 31:515–517, 1951
8. Liberson WT, Holmquest HJ, Scott D, et al: Functional electrotherapy: stimulation of the peroneal nerve synchronized with the swing phase of the gait of hemiplegic patients. Arch Phys Med Rehabil 42:101–105, 1961
9. Munsat TL, McNeal DR, Waters RL: Preliminary observations on prolonged stimulation of peripheral nerve in man. Recent Advances in Myology. Proceedings of the Third International Congress on Muscle Disuse, Newcastle upon Tyne, England, 1974, pp 42–50
10. Baker LL, Yeh C, Wilson D, et al: Electrical stimulation of wrist and fingers for hemiplegic patients. Phys Ther 59:1495–1499, 1979
11. Peckham PH, Mortimer JT, Marsolais EB: Alteration in the force and fatigability of skeletal muscle in quadriplegic humans following exercise induced by chronic electrical stimulation. Clin Orthop 114:326–334, 1976
12. Bowman BR, Baker LL, Waters RL: Positional feedback and electrical stimulation: an automated treatment for the hemiplegic wrist. Arch Phys Med Rehabil 60:497–502, 1979
13. Vodovnik L, Rebersek S: Improvements in voluntary control of paretic muscles due to electrical stimulation. In: Neural Organization and its Relevance to Prosthetics, eds. WS Fields, LA Leavitt. New York, Intercontinental Medical Book Corp, 1973, pp 101–116
14. Levine L, Knott M, Kabot H: Relaxation of spasticity of electrical stimulation of antagonist muscles. Arch Phys Med Rehabil 33:668–673, 1952
15. Vogel M, Weinstein L, Abramson A: Use of tetanizing current for spasticity. Phys Ther Rev 35:435–437, 1955
16. Dimitrijevic MR, Nathern DW: Studies of spasticity in man: 4. Changes in flexion reflex with repetitive cutaneous stimulation in spinal man. Brain 93:743–768, 1970
17. Stanic V, Acimovic-Jenezic R, Gross N, et al: Multichannel electrical stimulation for correction of hemiplegic gait. Scand J Rehabil Med 10:75–92, 1978
18. Rebersek S, Vodovnik L: Proportionally controlled functional electrical stimulation of hand. Arch Phys Med Rehabil 54:378–382, 1973
19. Gersh MR: Post-operative pain and transcutaneous electrical nerve stimulation. Phys Ther 58:1463–1466, 1978
20. Herman E: The use of transcutaneous nerve stimulation in the management of chronic pain. Physiotherapy (Canada) 29:65–71, 1977
21. Glenn WWL, Holcomb WG, Hogan SF, et al: Long-term stimulation of the phrenic nerve for diaphragm pacing. In: Functional Electrical Stimulation: Applications in Neural Prostheses, eds. FT Hambrecht, JB Reswick. New York, Marcel Dekker, 1977, pp 97–112
22. Friedman H, Nashold BS, Grimes J: Electrical Stimulation of the conus medullaris in the paraplegic—A five year review. In: Functional Electrical Stimulation: Applications in Neural Prostheses, eds. FT Hambrecht, JB Reswick. New York, Marcel Dekker, 1977, pp 173–183
23. Axelgaard J, McNeal DR, Brown JC: Lateral electrical surface stimulation for the

treatment of progressive scoliosis. Proceedings of the Sixth, International Symposium on External Control of Human Extremities, Dubrovnik, Yugoslavia, 1978, pp 63–70

24. Johnson DH, Thuston P, Ashcroft PJ: The Russian technique of faradism in the treatment of chondromalacia patellae. Physiotherapy (Canada) 29:266–268, 1977

25. Currier DP, Lehman J, Lightfoot P: Electrical stimulation in exercise of the quadriceps femoris muscle. Phys Ther 59:1508–1512, 1979

26. Munsat TL, McNeal DR, Waters RL: Effects of nerve stimulation on human muscle. Arch Neurol 33:608–617, 1976

27. Morris CJ, Salmons S: The innervation pattern of fast muscle fibers subjected to long-term stimulation. J Anat 120:412, 1975

28. Pette D: Coexistance of fast and slow type myosin light chains in single muscle fibers during transformation as induced by long-term stimulation. FEBS Lett, 83:128–130, 1977

29. Salmons S, Gale DR, Sreter FA: Ultrastructural aspects of the transformation of muscle fibre type by long-term stimulation: changes in Z lines and mitochondria. J Anat 127:17–31, 1978

30. Gracanin F: Use of functional electrical stimulation in rehabilitation of hemiplegic patients. Final report to HEW No. 19-P-58395-F-012-66, Ljubljana, Yugoslavia, 1972

31. Stefancic M, Rebersek S. Merletti R: The therapeutic effect of the Lubljana functional electronic peroneal brace. Europa Medicophysica 12:1–9, 1976

32. Gracanin F: The role of functional electrical stimulation of extremities in rehabilitation medicine. Europa Mediophysica 8:48–55, 1972

33. Ray CD: Electrical stimulation: new methods for therapy and rehabilitation. Scand J Rehab Med 10:65–74, 1978

34. Rancho Los Amigos Rehabilitation Engineering Center: Annual report of progress to the rehabilitation services administration. U.S. Department of Health, Education and Welfare, No. 8, 1979, pp 2–13, 24–25

35. Waters RL, McNeal DR, Perry J: Experimental correction of foot drop by electrical stimulation of the peroneal nerve. J Bone Joint Surg 57-A:1047–1054, 1975

36. Crastam B, Larson E, Previc T: Improvement of gait following functional electrical stimulation. Scand J Rehabil Med 9:7–13, 1977

37. Tang EL, McNeal DR, Kralj A, et al: Electrical stimulation and feedback training: effects on the voluntary control of paretic muscle. Arch Phys Med Rehabil, 57:228–233, 1976

38. Daves R. Gesink JW: Evaluation of electrical stimulation as a treatment for the reduction of spasticity. Bull Prosth Res 22:302–309, 1974

39. Lee W, McGovern JP, Duvall EN: Continuous tetanizing (low voltage) currents for relief of spasms. Arch Phys Med Rehabil 31:766–771, 1950

40. Strojnik P, Kralj A, Ursic I: Programmed six-channel electrical stimulator for complex stimulation of leg muscles during walking. IEEE Trans Biomed Eng 26:112–116, 1979

41. Kralj A, Trnkcozy A, Acimovic R: Improvement of locomotion in hemiplegic patients with multichannel electrical stimulation. Preceedings of Conference on Human Locomotor Engineering, University of Sussex, Brighton, England, 1970, pp 60–68

42. Bajd T, Kralj A, Sega J, et al: Two channel electrical stimulator providing standing of paraplegic patients. Phys Ther 61:526–527, 1981

43. Peckham PH, Mortimer JT: Restoration of hand function in the quadriplegic through electrical stimulation. In: Functional Electrical Stimulation: Applications in Neural Prosthesis, eds. FT Hambrecht, JB Reswick. New York, Marcel Dekker, 1977, pp 83–95

44. Case Western Reserve University Rehabilitation Engineering Center: second annual report of progress, 1978–1979, pp 15–18
45. Merletti R, Acimovic R, Grobelnik S, et al: Electrophysiological orthosis for the upper extremity in hemiplegia: feasibility study. Arch Phys Med Rehabil 56:507–513, 1975
46. Ranch Los Amigos Rehabilitation Engineering Center: annual report of progress to the rehabilitation services administration, U.S. Department of Health, Education and Welfare, No. 7, 1978, pp 2–12, 24–22
47. Ranch Los Amigos Rehabilitation Engineering Center: Annual report of progress to the rehabilitation services administration, US Department of Health, Education and Welfare, No. 6, 1977, pp 3–7, 15–18, 22–26
48. Hurd MM: Shoulder slings for hemiplegic: friend or foe? Arch Phys Med Rehabil 55:519–522, 1974
49. Benton LA, Baker LL, Bowman BR, et al: Functional electrical stimulation—a practical clinical guide. Rancho Los Amigos Rehabilitation Engineering Center, Downey, CA, 1980, pp 40–49, 55–106

3 Electromyography as a Clarifying Tool

Dean P. Currier

INTRODUCTION

Electromyography (*EMG*), simply and generically stated, is an electrophysiologic technique used to study the electrical activity of muscle or, more specifically, the motor units. EMG is applied in the study of muscle function during: biofeedback training; dynamic or static activities of sport, activities of daily living, and ergonomics; and in pathologic states of the musculoskeletal or neuromuscular systems. In medicine, electromyography is frequently referred to as clinical and diagnostic EMG.

The term *diagnostic EMG* has been a misnomer because electromyographic findings are not specific to any disease or disorder.[1] *Clinical EMG* may also be confusing, since EMG is used to differentiate between levels of motor unit activity in biofeedback training, and in various gaits, both of which are "clinical" uses of electromyography. To avoid misleading the reader, EMG for this discussion, is defined as the needle examination for differentiating from the normal state the status of peripheral nerve and skeletal muscle in myelopathies, neuropathies, and myopathies.

Historically, the needle technique of recording electrical activities of motor units by electronic methods was demonstrated by Adrian and Bronk in 1929.[2] The value of this method in medicine was reported in 1944 by Weddel, Feinstein, and Pattle.[3] Since World War II, the needle examination of EMG, along with nerve conduction studies, has been widely used to assist physicians in arriving at a diagnosis. Today EMG is appropriately used to gather information about the motor unit activity of muscle by the anatomist, ergonomist, kinesiologist, physical education specialist, physical therapist, physician, physiologist, and others.

This chapter contains an overview of the needle examination used to differentiate between the pathologic and normal state of muscle. The reader is cautioned that this information is an overview and to obtain a more thorough understanding of needle electromyography appropriate books on the subject must be consulted for the necessary detail.[4-8]

THE MOTOR UNIT

The *motor unit* is the functional unit of the neuromuscular system. It consists of a cell body (anterior horn cell), an axon (myelinated), neuromuscular junctions, and each muscle fiber is innervated by the terminal branches of the axon. In the muscle the axon of the motor unit divides into many terminal branches. Each terminal branch then innervates a muscle fiber. Muscle contains many motor units, but they vary according to the particular muscle. Feinstein and colleagues[9] reported that a single axon may innervate nine fibers in the external rectus, 25 fibers in the platysma, 108 fibers in the first lumbricale, and 1900 fibers in the gastrocnemius muscle. This variation in the innervation ratio of muscles will be reflected by the electrical activity seen on needle examination.

The individual fibers of a motor unit intermingle with fibers of other motor units in the muscle to provide a diffuse anatomic distribution. Muscle fibers of a single motor unit may not be in contact with other fibers of the same unit,[10] but are confined to a small area (5 to 20 mm) of muscle.[11]

Limb muscles receive their innervation from more than one spinal segment, and this is called *plurisegmental innervation.* Axons of the motor unit of a single muscle exit the spinal cord from two or more anterior nerve roots. A group of muscles supplied by one spinal segment is known as a *myotome.* Since limb muscles are innervated by two or more spinal segments, a muscle will have as many myotomes. For example, the triceps may be supplied by the C_{6-8}-T_1 myotomes and the medial head of the gastrocnemius by the S_{1-2} myotomes.

A synapse is formed between the terminal portion of an axon and its associated muscle fiber. The presynaptic ending of the axon contains acetylcholine, a transmitter substance, which is released when a nerve impulse is received. Once the acetylcholine is released from its storage vesicles, it interacts with the postsynaptic membrane (endplate) of the muscle fiber, resulting in an endplate potential. Quanta of acetylcholine are released about once per second when muscle is at rest. Although these amounts are too small to cause the muscle to contract, small transient depolarizations of the muscle fiber can be recorded as miniature endplate potentials. Only when many quanta of acetylcholine are released, is the amount and frequency of miniature endplate potentials sufficient to cause the muscle fiber to contract. The enzyme acetylcholinesterase, present in large amounts, hydrolyzes acetylcholine so that nerve impulses can be transmitted at high rates.[12, 13]

Motor Unit Potentials

Nerve and muscle cells have membranes that form a structural barrier and regulate metabolism. These membranes limit the movement of some ions, but permit others to diffuse freely across. This selective permeability creates a potential difference across the membrane so that at rest the cells are charged electrically. Thus, the membranes of nerves and muscles are excitable.

The potential difference is established by the unequal concentration of charged ions across the membrane. Sodium (Na^+) and chloride (Cl^-) ions are in higher concentration outside the cell (interstitial fluid), while potassium (K^+) and large protein (A^-) are in higher concentration inside the cell (intracellular fluid). The K^+ ions tend to leak or diffuse out of the cell into the interstitial fluid, while Na^+ ions tend to leak into the nerve and muscle cells. Because the membrane of a resting cell is more permeable to K^+ than to Na^+ ions, the concentrations of the ions change. This leakage of ions, particularly K^+, continues until the intracellular fluid reaches an electrically negative potential relative to the positive charge outside the cell. This leakage of ions contributes to the potential difference and when the dynamic equilibrium of the resting cell is reached, the condition created is the *resting membrane potential.* Thus, the resting potential exists in the resting cell because an active transport mechanism (sodium pump) keeps the intracellular concentration of Na^+ low, and the membrane maintains selective permeability. The membrane is more permeable to K^+ than to Na^+, but prevents the negative proteins from leaving the cell.

Energy necessary for the active transport mechanism and metabolism of the cells is obtained from the phosphate bonds of adenosinetriphosphate (ATP). Cells constantly use ATP to maintain their electrical equilibrium. They remain in equilibrium until some stimulus, such as a needle electrode or volitional command, reduces the potential across the membrane to a threshold level. The membrane is said to depolarize, causing excitation when its threshold level is reached.

The change in membrane potential brought about by a stimulus results in a brief electrical discharge known as an *action potential.* The action potentials recorded in needle electromyography are customarily described as motor unit potentials (MUPs). MUPs represent the electrical activity derived from muscle fibers of a motor unit(s). Since the muscle fibers of a single motor unit are intermingled in a muscle, they are distributed in time and space. Because of these temporal and spatial properties, the MUP recorded during the needle examination is a summated action of all potentials of the various muscle fibers of the particular unit. That is, the membranes of the various muscle fibers discharge electrically in sequence but at some distance apart. The needle electrode detects the temporal and spatial discharges as a summated signal or MUP. Figure 3-1 illustrates this phenomenon.

Note in Figure 3-1 that the action potential of the muscle fiber nearest the tip of the recording needle electrode is larger than the others. The recording electrode detects potential differences external to the muscle fibers and some distance from the source of the potentials. Because of the spatial relationship, the closer the potential is to the tip of the recording needle the larger it is and the greater its contribution to the size of the MUP. As the interstitial fluid surrounding nerve and muscle cells contain ions it is a good conducting medium. A *volume conductor* is a medium through which electrical activity will disperse so that a potential difference between active and inactive areas of muscle can be detected. Normal muscle

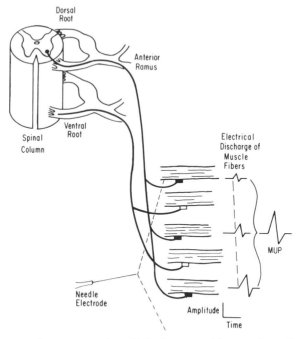

Fig. 3-1. Diagrammatic representation of plurisegmental innervation of muscle and of a summated motor unit potential recorded in needle electromyographic examinations. The dotted lines directed toward the needle represent volume conduction to the surrounding area and those joining the action potentials of individual muscle fibers represent temporal dispersion.

contractions, or pathologic muscle at rest or in states of activation serve as sources of electrical activity flowing through the volume of body fluid and electrolytes. Conductivity of bioelectric potentials through the volume conductor is not uniform because the area adjacent to muscle contains connective, vascular, and lipid materials that act as insulators. The results of variable volume conduction are displayed in the characteristics of the recorded MUPs. Each electrode placement will affect the size (amplitude), shape, and duration to some extent. Characteristics of normal MUPs will, however, fall within a range the electromyographer can use as a guide.

INSTRUMENTATION

Electromyography involves studying the electrical activity of MUPs by recording from muscle during graded contractions and at rest. The displayed electrical signals are summations of the individual action potentials from fibers of the motor unit(s) of the muscle being assessed. Several factors may, however, interfere with measurements of the activity of the specific muscle being examined. Such factors are caused by (1) volume conductions, which may result in display of potentials from nearby muscles; (2) disease or injury affecting a limited number or site of motor units of a muscle; and (3) the anatomic location of the muscle beneath other muscles. Because these factors may interfere with the recording and display of desired electrical signals, needle electrodes inserted directly into a selected muscle are essential for the electromyographic examination used for assessing neurologic diseases.

MUPs are very small (.01 to 4 mV) voltage discharges that must be detected, processed, and displayed. The electronic components or instruments used to measure the electrical phenomena of muscle and nerve constitute an instrumentation system. The basic instrumentation system (electromyograph) used to detect, process, and display motor unit potentials is comprised of electrodes, amplifiers, an oscilloscope, and a loud speaker. Accessories, such as a tape recorder, a delay line, storage oscilloscope, fiber optic recorder, signal averager, and cameras are often part of an electromyograph but will not be discussed in this overview.

Recording Electrodes

Since the electrical signal of motor units is directly available from the subject undergoing examination, it is transferred from the selected muscle to the electronic instrumentation system by two electrodes, which serve as conductors, linking the body to the electronic system. The ionic activity of various muscle states is transferred by electrodes in the form of electrical signals that are analogs or stimulations of motor unit activity. The transfer takes place at the muscle-electrode interface.

Surface electrodes applied to the overlying skin detect the global activity of muscle. The global activity of muscle can be recorded because surface electrodes usually have a greater than 50 mm^2 of focal point (leading off area) with the overlying skin. Since surface electrodes cannot detect single motor units, they are used only to record evoked muscle and nerve action potentials and to stimulate peripheral nerves in nerve conduction tests.

Needle electrodes are used when activity from a single or a few motor units is to be recorded. The focal points of needle electrodes are usually less than 1 mm^2 and can therefore detect a small area within a muscle.[14] Also, needle electrodes enable the electromyographer to examine muscles lying beneath others. Needle electrodes are usually very strong, stainless steel hypodermic needles that vary in length and diameter.

The distance separating the recording electrodes somewhat affects the magnitude of the MUP and its duration. For example, the duration of the recorded MUP is shorter with a hypodermic needle that contains two fine wires within its shell (bipolar) than with one that combines a single wire within its shell as the active electrode and the shell (concentric) as the reference electrode. If the distance between the active and the reference electrode is 0.5 mm the amplitude of the MUP is larger than it would be if the distance between them was 0.2 mm.[14]

The *monopolar electrode* is a solid stainless steel needle insulated with Teflon except at its tip, where it is bared for recording the electrical activity of motor units. Of the various needle electrodes available, the monopolar usually is the least uncomfortable for the patient because it has a small diameter and is insulated. The monopolar needle is the active or exploring electrode, while a surface disc, or another needle used concurrently, serves as an indifferent or reference electrode to complete the electric circuit. A separate metal plate, placed on the skin at some distance from the other two elements, serves as a ground.

Electric circuits require a source of power to drive current, a load in the form of resistors that require power, a source conductor or wire carrying the current to the load, and a conductor to return the current from the load to the source. If the return conductor or any object (e.g. chassis) is connected to the ground or earth, excess charges will be directed to the ground.[15] The result of this circuitry design is that the ground can neutralize charges so that the object has the same potential (zero) as the ground. The ground pathway has low resistance so that hazardous charges can be shunted to the ground before harm can occur. Patients are connected to electrical equipment and electrical equipment is connected to the ground. Thus, grounding serves as a safety measure and provides a zero potential. The latter helps in bioelectric recordings to reduce noises that would produce artifactual disturbances in the electrical signal being measured. A ground plate, usually larger than the electrodes, is used to record MUPs in the needle examination.

The *concentric needle electrode* consists of a hypodermic needle through which a fine wire is threaded. The fine wire is insulated from the shell of the steel needle and is exposed at the tip of the needle. The wire bared at the needle tip serves as the active electrode and measures the potential at its point of contact with muscle tissue. The shell (cannula) of the needle serves as the reference electrode. A separate metal plate placed on the skin at some distance from the concentric needle electrode serves as the ground.

The *bipolar needle electrode* contains two fine insulated wires imbedded within the lumen. Local electrical activity is measured between the two bare wire tips. The bipolar electrode may be larger in diameter than other needle electrodes but it has an advantage in that its shell serves as a ground; no additional metal plate is needed for grounding.

Sterilized needle electrodes must be free from contamination during the examination. Touching anything but the patient's cleansed skin is to be avoided. If the needle becomes contaminated, it must be discarded and a sterilized one used, otherwise a single needle is usually sufficient for the complete examination. For sterilization, the steam autoclave or gas methods are used. Personnel and facilities adept at sterilizing procedures for needle electrodes are available at hospitals and clinics and should be consulted. Steam autoclaving, however, usually consists of heating (121°–127 °C) at 1500–1800 mmHg pressure for 20 min. Ethyl oxide can be used for gas sterilization.

After the examination is completed, the needle is cleaned and carefully inspected for broken leads or bent tips and then sharpened with a sharpening stone. Electrodes may be cleaned electrically also.[14] Only concentric and bipolar needle electrodes can be resharpened. Monopolar electrodes have a very thin, soft insulation coating that is easily damaged when resharpening is attempted. The usual procedure is to destroy the needle when the tip is exposed excessively, or a break in the insulation or dullness occur.

Tips of needles should be inspected under a microscope and tested frequently with an ohmometer to determine impedance levels and electrical continuity. To test impedance place the monopolar needle tip in soft rubber or cork and immerse it in a container of saline. Connect the lead of the needle to one lead of the ohmometer and place the other terminal of the ohmmeter into the solution slowly. Concentric needle leads are connected to the ohmmeter and then immersed in saline for a reading. A reading of 25 to 30 megohms resistance is an indication the needle is faulty.

The Amplifier

Recorders and display devices must be compatible with the electrical signals of muscle. Because the electrical activity derived from the body is very small (microvolts and millivolts) and contains undesired signals, it must be conditioned and amplified. The *amplifier* is that part of the instrumentation system that conditions and amplifies the electrical output of the electrodes. The amplifier really consists of several separate amplifiers but is referred to as a single unit. Certain features of an amplifier are essential for processing and amplifying signals to be used in electromyography.

In most physiologic measurements desired and undesired interference signals are produced. The desired signal may be that of the motor unit(s) of a selected muscle, while the undesired interference signal (often called artifact or noise) may originate from several sources, either inside or outside the patient and is typically a 60-Hz signal. The *differential amplifier* accepts two input signals; it rejects the interference signal and amplifies the desired signal. The output signal is equal to the amplified difference between the two input signals.

Because the undesired interference signal appears between both the negative and positive inputs of the differential amplifier and ground in the same phase, it is called the *common mode signal.* The purpose of a differential amplifier is to reject common mode signals, which are expressed by the ratio between the amplitude (size) of the signal common to both inputs and to the amplitude difference between the inputs of an equivalent motor unit potential (differential signal). If a differential amplifier rejects two equal 1000 mV in-phase signals and amplifies a 1-mV out-of-phase signal, the amplifier has a *common mode rejection ratio* of 1000: 1. A high common mode rejection ratio is essential for rejecting interference from an electromyographic recording.

Distortion of motor unit potentials is, of course, undesirable. When electrodes and electrode tissue junctions are connected to an amplifier, high impedances are formed to reduce the size of the desired electrical signals. These undesired high impedances are minimized by making the input impedance of the amplifier many times greater than any impedance that could occur from the electrodes and metal-tissue junctions. *High input impedance* of the amplifier insures that little current is taken from the original motor unit signal to be amplified yet preserves the signal's voltage. This voltage will then be the only voltage amplified. Therefore, amplifiers should have an input impedance as high as possible to block undesired impedances and to minimize the amount of energy or power the amplifier has to provide to the recording system.

The motor unit signal contains various Fourier sine wave components as frequencies. The motor unit potentials of diseased muscle may have wave components as high as 10,000 Hz and very rapid transition phases between positive and negative portions of the waveform. The amplifier must have a *broad band frequency response;* that is, the frequency must range from 2 to 10,000 Hz.

The output size of a signal divided by its input size constitutes the *gain* of the amplifier. An amplifier must have sufficient voltage to operate other components of the system and to produce amplified signals large enough to be displayed. The gain of an amplifier is about 1000 when it produces a signal of 100 mV from an original signal of 0.1 mV on the oscilloscope. Amplifiers are limited to the size of signal (volts) that can be amplified. When zero volts are entering the amplifier, and the inputs are shorted (joined together), the output on the display will show some size to a produced signal or amplifier noise. This noise is, in addition to the interference signals caused by 60-Hz line current, fluorescent lights, diathermies, and poor grounds and is inherent in the design of the amplifier. Signals smaller than the amplifier noise cannot be distinguished from it.

The Display Unit

The *oscilloscope* permits visual display of motor unit potentials after they are processed and amplified. It consists of a cathode ray tube (picture tube) with external controls that change the characteristics of the display to suit the desired measurement requirements. The electron beam of the oscilloscope has a very small mass and inertia, enabling it to respond to and display instantaneous electrical signals as well as very high frequency waveforms. The oscilloscope does not provide a permanent record. The signal, however, can be delayed a few seconds for visual inspection or for recording by devices.

The Audiomonitor

The electrical signals of skeletal muscle vacillate according to the abnormal conditions of its fibers and nerve supply. These vacillations occur at frequencies within the range of sound audible to humans. The changes in sound can be amplified and fed to a loud speaker for listening. If the audioamplifier and loud speaker are interfaced with the oscilloscope, the examiner can listen to the sounds of various waveforms concurrent with their visual display. Audio and visual input are helpful to the examiner in recognizing particular signals associated with normal and abnormal muscle and nerve. The audioamplifier must be capable of amplifying signals within the frequency range found in muscle (2 to 10,000 Hz).

NORMAL MOTOR UNIT CHARACTERISTICS

The motor unit potential is the primary objective of the needle examination. Departure from the traits of so-called "normal" motor unit activity serves as a basis for recognizing the abnormal electrical activity of diseased or injured muscle. The traits of normal motor units, like those of abnormal potentials, follow specific patterns when examined under selected conditions.

Whenever a needle is inserted into muscle, it pierces the cell membranes of the muscle fibers. The injured cell produces a spontaneous burst of electrical discharges because the inserted needle mechanically stimulates the membrane. The burst of discharges (called injury potentials) or *insertion activity* ceases instantaneously, when movement of the needle insertion stops. The duration of the insertion activity of normal muscle averages less than 300 ms.[5] Insertion activity also occurs when the needle electrode is shifted from one location to another in the relaxed muscle, and in normal muscle may have amplitudes as great as 2 mV.

Occasionally, when the needle electrode is inserted into the middle region of a muscle, small spontaneous potentials of up to 2 ms duration and 100 μV in amplitude appear on the oscilloscope.[7] These potentials sound similar to seashell noise and are high frequency, monophasic, negatively shaped waves. They are called *endplate potentials*. The needle disrupts a small number of vesicles of acetylcholine causing the endplate potentials to discharge randomly and independently of nerve impulses, thus no muscle contraction results. These potentials can be mistaken for fibrillation potentials if the initial negative phases are not observed.

Nerve potentials are also observed in the motor endplate regions of muscle. Like endplate potentials, the nerve potentials are small (20 to 200 μV in amplitude) and of short duration (1 to 3 ms). They are diphasic in waveform with an initial negative phase, and repeat at a rate of 20 to 100/s.[8] A distinguishing feature is that the patient feels sharp pain as the nerve potential occurs but the pain is immediately relieved when the position of the needle electrode is changed. Nerve potentials represent discharges from very small nerve branches, which are penetrated by the needle electrode. Their characteristic "rushing" noise is similar to that of seashell sounds.

No electrical activity is derived from normal muscle (or at least cannot be seen on an oscilloscope with presently designed amplifiers) during rest (relaxation). The baseline should appear as a straight horizontal line of electrons traversing the fluorescent grid of the oscilloscope with each sweep. This condition is called *electrical silence*. Actually, some amplifier noise—hissing—may be heard, but no deflections of the baseline occur when muscle is resting.

Motor unit potentials are the chief attraction recorded from muscle during voluntary contraction. During muscle contraction, the fibers in a single motor unit contract asynchronously. This asynchronous contraction causes slight differences in the time each action potential arrives near the tip of the needle electrode to result in a summated motor unit potential. If the electrode tip is located at the point at which the MUP originates, the initial phase will be negative, otherwise it is positive. Most normal MUPs have three phases, with the initial phase being positive.

(Note: electrophysiologists orient the upward deflection of an action potential negatively on the oscilloscope. Proper connection of the negative and positive electrode leads to the amplifier is necessary for this orientation.)

The shape, duration, amplitude, and rates of discharge vary in different muscles. The configuration of normal unit potentials may not exceed four phases. A phase is determined each time the wave touches or crosses the baseline. Some normal motor unit potentials are jagged and appear to have several phases but these jagged occurrences do not approximate, touch, or cross the baseline. About 10 to 12 percent of MUPs may have more than four phases (polyphasic) but are considered within normal limits if their numbers do not exceed 15 percent. Exceptions include the deltoid, which receives hypodermic injections, and the extensor digitorum brevis, which is constantly irritated by shoes. These events may account for the polyphasic potentials that occur frequently in these muscles.

A normal MUP has a duration that ranges between 3 and 15 ms and has an amplitude of 100 to 4000 uV. The rate at which the MUP is discharged depends on the strength of muscle contraction but occurs between 3 and 30/s. Over the loudspeaker, MUPs sound like sharp thumps.

As the strength of muscular contraction is voluntarily increased, additional motor units are recruited. Recruitment continues with graduated contractions so that during a very strong or maximum muscle contraction, motor unit potentials become superimposed on each other to obliterate the oscilloscope grid. This situation, called the *interference* or *recruitment* pattern, when present makes it impossible to distinguish individual traits of motor unit potentials. The superimposed potentials result in increased amplitudes that should not be confused with giant motor units (see below). With maximum recruitment, the sound of individual MUPs change from sharp thumps to a roar.

Recording with different needle electrodes will affect the traits of motor unit potentials slightly; that is, different amplitudes and durations are obtained with monopolar, concentric, and bipolar needle electrodes because their leading-off areas vary as the strength of muscle contraction is voluntarily increased.

ABNORMAL MOTOR UNIT CHARACTERISTICS

In neuromuscular disease spontaneous electrical activity of clinical value, other than nerve and endplate potentials, may occur when the muscle is relaxed. Abnormal electrical activity also occurs during voluntary muscle contraction. Several varieties of abnormal electrical activity can be identified in neuromuscular disease and injury.

Insertion activity is often easily induced and prolonged in muscle that is denervated or affected by diseases such as myotonia and poliomyositis. Occasional positive sharp waves (see below) are seen as insertional activity in denervated muscle. Insertional potentials are prolonged when the activity continues after the needle has stopped moving. Prolonged insertional activity is a very subjective finding and should be confirmed by several additional insertions in the same muscle. Prolonged insertional activity or irritability may often be the only abnormal finding in radiculopathies. Insertional activity may also be diminished or absent when muscular atrophy is present or when the number of excitable muscle fibers is reduced. The diminished insertional activity is proportional to the extent of muscle tissue reduction.[4]

Fibrillation potentials are small spontaneous potentials that appear when muscle is at rest, or after voluntary muscle contractions. Fibrillation potentials can be facilitated by heating the affected muscle and by moving the needle electrode, thus providing mechanical irritation. Although fibrillation potentials are seen rarely in healthy muscle, they are considered abnormal and are recognized with certainty by their characteristic short durations (about 2 ms or less) of initial positive deflection, and high-pitched click (likened to wrinkling cellophane or to raindrops on the roof).[4] Their waveform may be diphasic or triphasic. The diphasic waveform usually occurs when potentials are recorded in the endplate regions and are difficult to distinguish from the miniature endplate potentials with their initial negative deflection.[5] The amplitude of fibrillation potentials is also small and ranges from about 10 to 300 μV. Their appearance is usually irregular, with discharges of from 1 to 30/s. Fibrillation potentials are often reported using a scheme of grades. One such scheme is presented in Table 3-1. Fibrillation potentials are found in neuropathies, myelopathies, and myopathies. Their origin is uncertain and they are usually numerous in acute neurologic processes but subside as neurons are reinnervated. Fibrillations are occasionally visible in the tongue.

Positive sharp waves are descriptive because they appear with a characteristic sharp initial positive deflection. They are usually monophasic but can be diphasic, with the negative deflection appearing as a slow decay following the sharp positive deflection. Their duration may vary greatly (2 to 100 ms) but usually last from 10 to 20 ms. Amplitudes of these waves vary greatly from 20 to 4000 uV. A dull thud may describe their sound as they appear spontaneously and irregularly between 2 and 100 times per second. The average discharge frequency of positive sharp waves is 10/s. Positive sharp waves are believed to originate from or be related to irritation of injured, single muscle fibers. They are not seen in healthy muscle and often accompany fibrillation potentials in frequency and pattern. Although positive sharp waves are most frequently associated with denervated muscle, they are found in myelopathies and myopathies.

Fasciculation potentials are spontaneously occurring contractions of groups of muscle fibers in healthy and abnormal muscle. Because fasciculations are representative of a group or bundle of muscle fibers, they are visible as muscle twitches.

TABLE 3-1. Scheme for grading fibrillation potentials

Grade	Description
0	No fibrillation potentials observed
+	Fibrillation activity noted upon needle insertion or movement (may be equivocal)
++	A few fibrillation potentials noted in each of several samplings
+++	Many fibrillation potentials noted in several but not all samplings
++++	Many fibrillation potentials in all samplings

(Data from Rodriquez AA and Oester YT: Fundamentals of electromyography. In: Electrodiagnosis and Electromyography, 3rd. edn., ed. Licht S. Baltimore, Waverly Press.)

Benign fasciculations are seen in healthy muscles over much of the body but are more commonly seen in the hand and foot muscles, and in the gastrocnemius muscle as cramps. Fasciculations are seen during needle examinations as pathologic potentials in myelopathies and neuropathies. They may be observed in benign myokymia, nerve root compressions, and inflammations, and occasionally in peripheral nerve injuries. These potentials have significant value when found in conditions involving the anterior horn cell, such as motor neuron disease, syringomyelia, poliomyelitis, spinal muscular atrophy, and amyotrophic lateral sclerosis.

The spontaneously occurring fasciculation potentials are often difficult to distinguish from the normal motor unit potentials because their amplitude (5 to 1200 uV), duration (5 to 25 ms), and waveform are often similar. Fasciculation potentials appear as di-, or triphasic or complex (four or more phases) forms. The complex or polyphasic forms are more frequently found in pathologic fasciculations. Their rate is usually slow, less than 1/s. They produce a sharp thumping sound, which may be heard as low and rough.[8]

In motor neuron or anterior-horn cell diseases motor unit potentials may have increased amplitudes and durations. Peripheral sprouting from surviving axons that hook up with denervated adjacent muscle fibers results in enlargement of the motor unit territory and an increase in fiber density.[8] The enlarged potentials are called *giant motor unit potentials* and can exceed 5 mV in amplitude. The rate at which the giant units fire is slow and irregular, often resembling normal MUPs.

In a single motor unit the muscle fibers discharge in an almost synchronous fashion, but because they spread out at a given area the recorded potential appears summated as a diphasic or triphasic waveform. Disease or injury may destroy some muscle fibers in one or several motor units, resulting in temporal changes. These temporal changes give a recorded motor unit potential the appearance of an asynchronous discharge. This type of discharge results in a motor unit potential that is either complex or has several phases. A *polyphasic* or *complex potential* represents such a motor unit, and may be indicative of degeneration or regeneration of muscle fiber innervation. It has more than five phases (5 to 25), which often prolong its duration (2 to 25 ms). The asynchronous discharge causes a rough, rasping sound on the audiomonitor of the EMG unit. Polyphasic potentials are recognized during weak voluntary muscular contractions and occur in neuropathies, myelopathies, and myopathies. They occur in healthy muscle and may account for as much as 10 percent of the motor unit potentials seen on the oscilloscope. Polyphasic potentials may also be associated with fasciculations and giant motor unit potentials to provide varied ranges of amplitude (20 to 5000 uV) and frequency (less than 1 to 30/s).

High frequency discharges that defy characteristic description may be seen in neuropathies, myelopathies, and myopathies. They are usually brief bursts of electrical discharges that start and stop abruptly and may be facilitated by movement of the needle electrode. The distinguishing features of high frequency discharges include: fast rate of discharge; varying amplitudes; and bizarre configurations. High frequency discharges are usually seen in resting muscle.

TABLE 3-2. Summary of electrophysiologic characteristics of abnormal motor unit potentials

Waveform	Amplitude (μv)	Duration (ms)	Number of peaks
Fibrillation	10 to 300	≲2	Di- or triphasic; positive initial deflection
Positive sharp wave	20 to 4000	2 to 100	Mono- or diphasic
Fasciculation	5 to 1200	5 to 25	Five or less
Polyphasic	20 to 5000	2 to 25	Five or more

(Data from Rodriquez AA and Oester YT: Fundamentals of electromyography. In: Electro-diagnosis and Electromyography 3rd. edn., ed. Licht S. Baltimore, Waverly Press, 1971.)

High frequency discharges associated with the myotonias are more characteristic than other high frequency activity. These discharges increase in frequency (10 to 150 Hz) and then decrease in rate to cause wax and wane sounds (changing pitch) like a "divebomber." They are called *myotonic discharges* or *potentials*. They appear when the needle electrode is inserted into a muscle affected by myotonia and may continue to discharge for several seconds. Slight movement of the needle or tapping the affected muscle usually triggers the myotonic discharges. These discharges may be related to an unstable muscle membrane.

Table 3-2 summarizes the electrophysiologic characteristics of abnormal motor unit potentials.

THE NEEDLE EXAMINATION

The needle examination is used to determine the functional status of the motor unit by measuring and interpreting the electrical activity within a muscle. Various sites along the pathway of the motor unit can be affected by disease or injury to cause abnormal electrical activity. These sites include, in descending order, the anterior horn cell, the spinal nerve root, the plexus, the nerve branch, the neuromuscular junction, and the muscle fibers.

The electromyographer must possess a thorough knowledge of anatomy, physiology, neuromuscular pathology, kinesiology, electronic instrumentation, and the interpretation of various forms of abnormal electrical activity. A history and a neurologic examination prior to needle examination are essential. Familiarization with the patient's medical record is also helpful.

Preparation of the Patient

The patient must be psychologically and physically prepared for the needle examination. A brief explanation of the procedures will help prepare the subject psychologically. Because the examination involves measurement of motor unit potentials by inserting a needle into muscles, the patient must be informed of this and be assured that every precaution will be taken to minimize his discomfort. The patient's cooperation throughout the examination is necessary. Positioning the patient supine or in a semireclining position with the use of a treatment table, pillows, and sandbags will help to relax him or her. Undue attention should not be given to the process of inserting needles. Sometimes use of the word "pins" rather than needles and telling the patient that he can see the activity on TV helps his attitude toward the examination.

Placement of Electrodes

After the patient is psychologically and physically prepared for the needle examination, the electrodes can be positioned. The muscle to be examined should be identified and palpated. The skin should then be thoroughly cleansed with alcohol or a solution recommended by local medical review groups. Place the reference electrode near the location to be explored. The reference electrode depends on the type of exploring needle selected. The ground electrode should be placed over bone or tendons near the muscle or muscles to be examined, after electrode jelly has been applied. If several muscles of the upper extremity are to be examined for example, the ground electrode can be secured over the olecranon process of the humerus. Skin resistance can be reduced greatly if the electrode jelly is massaged into the skin in addition to being applied over the surface. Tape or rubber strapping will be sufficient for securing the ground electrode, assuming proper preparation has been made and all electrodes are connected to the amplifiers via the connecting cable. The exploring needle is then ready for insertion and start of the examination.

Needle Insertion

The muscle under examination should be relaxed. A quick plunge of the inserting needle held at a right angle to the muscle will cause minimum discomfort to the patient. After the needle is inserted into the selected muscle of a relaxed patient to a depth of a few centimeters, electrical silence of the baseline should be observed along with only amplifier noise (hissing sound) on the audiomonitor. The electromyographer may hold onto the "handle" of the needle electrode as long as he does not move it. Such movement will mechanically stimulate the fiber membranes and may result in depolarization of muscle fibers.

Examination Procedure

Additional instruction to the patient at this time is helpful. The clinician may suggest that the patient relax. He should also be informed that the needle will move from time to time, and that he should contract the muscle on command. The needle should now be moved enough to evoke insertion activity and provide visual observation. If the response is questionable, the procedure should be repeated. The patient should be asked to contract the muscle weakly, then observe; contract moderately strong, then observe; contract maximally while providing resistance, then observe. The patient can relax the contracted muscle once the clinician is sure of the motor unit activity (amplitude, duration, shape, frequency, and recruitment pattern) observed during the various conditions. The observation and contraction procedures are repeated by advancing the needle to a greater depth than during the previous observation. After two or three depths are explored, the needle can be withdrawn to the original depth, avoiding excessive withdrawal from muscle and skin. The exploring needle can rapidly be inserted at a new angle and depth to examine a different portion of the muscle. Different techniques of needle insertions have been used to examine a muscle. If the clinician thinks of the muscle as a dial of a clock or compass, the needle can be inserted diagonally to 12, 3, 6 or 9 o'clock positions or north, east, south, and west, respectively. At each location three successive depths can be studied. This totals 15 sites of examination within the muscle before the needle is completely withdrawn.

The controls of the electromyographic unit must be manually altered whenever the motor unit potentials are so large as to consume the grid of the oscilloscope and likewise when the potentials are very small. Suggested control settings of the amplifier might be 100 μV per division at rest and perhaps 200 μV per division during maximum voluntary contraction. The sweep speed of the oscilloscope should be set at 10 ms per division and increased and decreased according to needs.

Once the exploring electrode has been withdrawn from a muscle, it is held in the hand of the electromyographer while another area is prepared for muscle insertion. The exploring needle electrode is inserted into another prepared muscle and is advanced by steps to three depths and five sites (15 total sites). In each location of the exploring electrode, observations are made of the particular electrical activity. After each muscle is examined, the data observed are recorded on a form. The electromyographer plans the various steps of the needle examination and modifies them as the information develops. Muscles are selected according to the patient's problems. For this reason, no routine procedure for examining specific muscles is necessary. The patient's history and physical findings serve as a guide. The examination may last a few or many minutes, but 1 h is usually the maximum that a patient can comfortably tolerate. The patient should be rescheduled if additional time is required.

POTENTIALS ENCOUNTERED IN DISEASE AND INJURY

The EMG needle examination is of considerable value in differentiating various problems involving the neuromuscular system. Descriptions of normal and abnormal characteristics of motor unit potentials have been presented. Since the electrical characteristics of the motor unit change in disease and injury states, specific EMG findings can aid in differentiating between disease and injury states. The reader must realize that abnormal motor unit potentials are not characteristic of specific disease entities or diagnosis within a grouping; some abnormal potentials can be found among all disease groupings. Each grouping can, however, be differentiated from another by combinations of findings and by characteristics peculiar to a specific grouping. Experienced electromyographers can further differentiate between conditions within a grouping or subgrouping by using information derived from the patient's history, clinical examination, nerve conduction tests, and findings from the needle examination. Three broad groupings will be considered: myelopathies, neuropathies, and myopathies.

Myelopathies

This grouping includes conditions effecting the anterior horn cells in the spinal cord. Such conditions include: spinal tumors, syringomyelia, poliomyelitis, spinal muscular atrophy (Werdnig-Hoffman and Kugelberg-Welander syndromes), amyotrophic lateral sclerosis, nerve root compressions, and others.

Abnormal electrical findings possible within this grouping include: prolonged insertion activity; fasciculations; fibrillations; positive sharp waves and decreased numbers of motor units (decreased recruitment); increased amplitude and durations (giant MUPs) of potentials; and polyphasic potentials. The rate at which the motor unit potentials are discharged may or may not be decreased. Variations occur with the severity of the condition.

Pathology of the anterior horn cells is usually compatible with findings of some of the abnormal electrical activity described but with normal motor and sensory nerve conduction tests as well. Finding fasciculations and giant motor unit potentials strongly point to pathology of the anterior horn cells. These potentials frequently are seen in diseases of the anterior horn cells and their absence make it difficult to clarify motor neuron problems.

Spinal muscular atrophy involves muscle patterns similar to those seen in muscular dystrophy; that is, weakness may begin in proximal muscles of the legs, in muscles of the pelvic area, or in a diffuse fashion. The disorder may begin in childhood or adolescence and progress slowly to degeneration of motor neurons of the spinal cord. Electrical activity of affected musculature on needle examination may consist of fibrillation potentials, positive sharp waves, polyphasic potentials, fasciculations, and giant motor unit potentials. The recruitment pattern is often reduced on maximum voluntary effort. Bizarre high frequency discharges are occasionally seen.

Another motor neuron disease seen in the EMG laboratory is *amyotrophic lateral sclerosis.* This disease causes degeneration of corticospinal tracts, resulting in weakness of muscles in the upper and lower extremities. Spontaneous electrical activity is often found in affected muscles in the form of prolonged insertional activity, fibrillation potentials, positive sharp waves, and fasciculations. Polyphasic potentials as well as decreased recruitment of motor units can be found in muscle contraction. Giant motor units with long durations are also found.

Patients with acute *poliomyelitis* are uncommon today, but the condition is occasionally seen in the EMG laboratory. Individuals who have had poliomyelitis may develop symptoms resembling amyotrophic lateral sclerosis.[16] The symptoms of muscle atrophy apparently progress slowly. Findings on needle examination are similar to those described for motor neuron disorders.

Spinal tumors often reveal EMG findings compatible with denervation, confined to segmental distributions of one or a few nerves. The needle examination is aimed at careful exploration of several muscles having different segmental distributions to locate the tumor. The EMG findings are similar to those expected of denervation.

Nerve root compression of the spinal cord is often the result of prolapsed intervertebral discs. The compression places pressure on the nerve root at the segmental level of the prolapsed disc. When muscles are examined in an orderly fashion by needle electrode, the lesion can be located accurately. Several myotomes should be examined. Often, positive sharp waves and prolonged insertional activity constitute the only abnormal electrical activity. A large number of polyphasic potentials may be seen along with fasciculations, fibrillation potentials, and bizarre high frequency discharges. The paravertebral musculature must always be explored when a myelopathy is suspected. Several muscles of a particular myotome with abnormal electrical findings help to establish a prolapsed intervertebral disc problem. Abnormal electrical findings of a single muscle may be insufficient evidence to support the claim of a disc disorder.

Neuropathies

Peripheral nerves are subject to various disorders, including inflammatory, hereditary, toxic, nutritional, metabolic, entrapment and compression, and traumatic causes. The disorders can produce a wide variety of clinical signs and symptoms because of the mixed motor and sensory components of involved autonomic and peripheral nervous system components. Electromyography is of great value in this group of disorders, especially when the peripheral nerves have damage to their myelin, axonal breakdown, and compression located at or distal to the level of their spinal roots.

Damage to the motor units may result in weakness, paralysis, decreased or absent deep tendon reflexes, and muscle atrophy. Electrically, abnormal motor unit potentials fluctuate greatly in denervation because of varying degrees of damage. Polyphasic potentials are frequently seen in neuropathies. The presence of increased insertion activity, fibrillations, fasciculation potentials, positive sharp waves, and bizarre high frequency activity are helpful, along with the slowing of motor and sensory nerve conduction velocities, in providing evidence of a neuropathy. The single most common finding in the needle examination that may aid in differentiating neuropathies from myelopathies and myopathies, and in assessing the degree of involvement is the decreased or partial interference (recruitment) pattern observed with maximum voluntary muscular contraction. Whereas maximum voluntary muscle contractions produce recruitment patterns that obliterate the oscilloscope grid, defective motor units drop out or cannot discharge with maximum effort by creating gaps in the electrical pattern.

Damage to the sensory nerve fibers may cause decreased sensation and decreased or absent deep tendon reflexes. Injury to the autonomic nerve fibers result in loss of anhidrosis (sweating), vasomotor tone, and possible loss of hair, dry skin and brittle nails.

Injuries and disease of somatic nerves can be classified into subgroups, such as compression injuries, traumatic conditions, and peripheral neuropathies.

Compression of nerves often involves only one nerve or a single spinal segment. Root compression may be due to prolapsed intervertebral discs or extramedullary tumors. Clinically, symptoms can include decreased deep tendon reflexes and sensation, but pain, temperature, and tactile sensation usually continue to be perceived by the patient. Although nerve conduction tests are usually normal in *radiculopathy,* the needle examination may reveal one or more signs of abnormal motor unit activity including: increased insertional activity, increased frequency of polyphasic potentials, fasciculations, fibrillation potentials, positive sharp waves, and bizarre high frequency activity.

Thoracic outlet syndrome may be the result of compression of the subclavian artery, or the lower roots or cord of the brachial plexus. Patients with this syndrome may complain of intermittent, deep aching pain or paresthesia along the distribution of the ulnar nerve. The pain is often increased by raising the affected arm. Conduction tests and needle examination of muscles innervated by the ulnar nerve are mostly unrewarding. Study of the F-wave traits may be helpful in evaluating this condition.

Major peripheral nerves, such as the median, ulnar, and radial of the upper extremities, and the peroneal, femoral, and posterior tibial nerves of the lower extremities are subject to *entrapment* at specific locations along their paths. A variety of causes result in these syndromes. Depending on the severity of the condition, needle examinations may or may not provide confirmatory data of partial denervation in muscles innervated by the affected nerve. Compression or entrapments of peripheral nerves often do not result in sufficient damage to cause denervation. Nerve conduction tests are usually the most rewarding portion of the electrophysiologic examination.

Traumatic injury of peripheral nerves can be caused directly by gun shot or knife wounds, by accidental stretch at birth, or from falls and vehicular accidents. Lesions often involve the nerve plexuses or individual major peripheral nerves. Needle examination findings are compatible with those outlined for diseases and injuries of somatic nerves proportional to the severity of the condition being assessed. The *peripheral neuropathies* are the most widely varied disorders of this grouping of diseases and injuries of somatic nerves. Damage to the axon, myelin, and connective tissue of peripheral nerves result.

Hereditary-familial conditions may include peroneal muscular atrophy (Charcot-Marie-Tooth disease) and hypertrophic interstitial neuropathy (Dejerine-Scottas disease). The former disease resembles a myelopathy in that fasciculations and giant motor unit potentials may be found along with other neuropathic findings including: fibrillations, many polyphasic potentials, and bizarre high-frequency activity. Distinguishing features of peroneal muscular atrophy are the clinical findings and marked slowing of motor nerve conduction velocities. In hypertrophic interstitial neuropathy the thickened peripheral nerves are easily palpated, the nerve conduction velocity is slowed greatly, and the needle examination may reveal reduced recruitment patterns and giant motor unit potentials. This condition often results in peripheral nerves having an excessively high threshold to electrical stimulation.[7]

An *inflammatory condition* involving mostly spinal roots and peripheral nerves is *Guillain-Barré syndrome* (active infectious polyradiculoneuritis). Patients who have this syndrome show paralysis of sudden onset, starting in the feet and ascending to the trunk, shoulders, and face. Respiratory and swallowing difficulties may occur. Needle examinations of affected muscles may reveal reduced recruitment patterns and polyphasic potentials. Fibrillation potentials often follow the onset of this syndrome in about 2 weeks. Nerve conduction velocity is usually slowed diffusely along the course of the nerve,[7] but occasionally no changes in velocity are noted in the acute phase.[8]

Alcoholic polyneuropathy, pellagra, and *vitamin B$_{12}$ neuropathy* are examples of nutritional disorders. Alcoholic polyneuropathy is the most common of the above nutritional conditions seen in the EMG laboratory. Needle examination findings often include polyphasic and fibrillation potentials, positive sharp waves, and reduced recruitment patterns, particularly in distal muscles of the extremities. Nerve conduction measurements are often abnormal.

Vascular and metabolic etiologies have been labeled as contributing factors to the common neuropathy that results from *diabetes mellitus.* Sensory fibers seem to be affected more than motor nerve fibers, which lead to the frequent abnormal sensory nerve conduction traits. The nerves of the lower extremities appear to be involved more often than those of the upper extremities.[5] Polyphasic and fibrillation potentials and positive sharp waves may be found upon needle examination but are not specific since these are found in most peripheral neuropathies.

Metals such as lead, mercury and arsenic are *toxic* to the peripheral nerves. The distally located nerves often undergo demyelination and degeneration, which ultimately result in foot and wrist drop, anesthesia of the glove-stocking type, decreased or absent deep tendon reflexes, and paresthesias. Motor nerve conduction usually slows in the upper extremities, while fibrillation potentials and positive sharp waves may be found on EMG assessment.[6]

Myopathies

Myopathies are diseases of muscle and can be separated into genetic, acquired, endocrine, metabolic, parasitic, and myotonic disorders.[7] Only the most common disorders of muscle are considered here. *Genetic muscular disorders* include the dystrophies of Duchenne, facioscapulohumeral, limb-girdle, and distal muscular types. *Acquired myopathy* includes polymyositis, while the *endocrine type* is represented by Addison disease and Cushing syndrome. McArdle disease and periodic paralysis are *metabolic myopathies* and trichinosis is a parasitic muscular disease. Myotonia includes several varieties that are usually considered by themselves. Myasthenia gravis and botulism, involving a defect in neuromuscular transmission in which acetylcholine is destroyed prematurely by cholinesterase, are included in this grouping.

The primary defect in myopathies seems to occur in muscle fibers with random muscle cell destruction. Motor units affected by these diseases have a progressive decreasing number of muscle fibers. The nerve innervation that permits surviving muscle fibers within any motor unit to function normally, is spared. The electromyographic effect of muscle disease is that less tension is exerted by a given motor unit and the temporal and spatial characteristics of that unit are decreased. In effect then, the muscles are weak and the motor units seen in recruitment patterns on needle examination are reduced in size (amplitude) and duration because large numbers of deteriorated fibers in the motor units discharge on maximum voluntary effort and are doing so at faster rates and in greater numbers than normal units would for a given amount of tension. Although certain electrical findings can differentiate myopathies from myelopathies and neuropathies, no particular EMG activity differentiates the various types of muscle disease, except for the myotonias.

Distrophies involve loss of muscle cells, to varying degrees, causing muscular weakness, atrophy leading to paralysis, and decreased or absent deep tendon reflexes. Many of the varieties of muscular dystrophy are X-linked. Some effect males, while others effect both males and females. The dystrophies are both malignant and benign in their progression. Needle examination of the dystrophies could reveal: full recruitment on maximum contraction but with reduced amplitude, prolonged insertional activity, decreased duration of motor unit potentials (1 to 3 ms) increased numbers of polyphasic potentials, fibrillation potentials, positive sharp waves. and bizarre high frequency activity. Nerve conduction tests are within normal limits.

Polymyositis appears as nonsupportive inflammatory changes associated with connective tissue disorders resulting in tenderness and pain, and in muscular weakness.[5, 7] Some patients with polymyositis have associated skin lesions. Needle examination may reveal prolonged insertional activity, fibrillation potentials, and bizarre high frequency activity.

In *endocrine myopathies* proximal muscle wasting and weakness occur. Extraocular muscles may be involved in hyperthyroidism. EMG changes may include one or more of the characteristic myopathic, abnormal motor unit traits.

Periodic paralysis is a transient muscular paralysis associated with a disturbance of potassium, which may be secondary to renal disease, and hypokalemia. Another type is familial and inherited, with autosomal dominance, and hyperkalemia. During mild occurrences, the needle examination is likely to show a marked decrease in the recruitment pattern, and single unit potentials may be of short duration. When the condition is severe enough to result in muscular paralysis, the EMG examination reveals electrical silence, which is seen at rest in healthy tissue. The hyperkalemic variety of periodic paralysis differs from the hypokalemic type in EMG findings by the occurrence of spontaneous activity, such as prolonged insertional activity, fibrillation potentials, and myotonic-like discharges at rest. These potentials may become more prominent during an acute episode. Motor unit potentials are reduced in number and are of short duration on voluntary contraction.[7]

McArdle syndrome, like periodic paralysis, is a form of metabolic myopathy caused by a deficiency in muscle phosphorylase. Lactate or pyruvate do not accumulate following exercise. EMG findings are normal, but if performed during muscle cramping after exercise, electrical silence can be expected. Electrical stimulation at 18 pps produces a quick decrement in the size of the evoked potentials.[17]

The patient with a *myotonic disorder* has difficulty performing rapidly alternating movements (adiadochokinesia) because muscle is slow to relax after voluntary contraction or after electrical and mechanical stimulation. This condition has been attributed to a problem involving the muscle cell membrane. Clinically, the myotonic disorders can be divided into several forms, such as congenita, dystrophy, paradoxa, acquisitia, and paramyotonia.[7] All forms are inherited and familial but have different characteristics. Needle examination reveals myopathic activity during voluntary muscular contractions. The distinguishing electrical feature of the myotonias is the so-called "myotonic discharges" when the muscle being examined by the needle, percussion, or following voluntary contraction, is stimulated. Myotonic discharges are described as high frequency potentials that rise (wax) to about 100 pps and then suddenly decrease in frequency (wane) and amplitude. The rise and fall of these potentials produce unique audible sounds described as a "divebomber," which gradually subside to silence as the stimulation or effort ceases.

Myasthenia gravis, although a disease of neuromuscular transmission, is grouped as a myopathy in this discussion. An insufficient quantity of acetylcholine or an excessive amount of cholinesterase has the effect of decreasing motor unit potentials of muscle fibers. Muscular fatigue results faster than normal with repeated movements, depending, of course, on the severity of the disease. Needle examination of affected muscles will reveal normal motor unit activity. Careful examination of affected muscles may reveal a pattern of decrement in the amplitudes of the motor unit potentials with continued weak contraction. An electrophysiologic study of the condition by applying electrical stimulation at varying pulse rates, is most rewarding.

Reporting the Examination

A prepared form should be used during the needle examination for the examiner's convenience. The form should provide space and lined divisions for identifying the patient; date of examination; the names of muscles examined and their nerve supply; and for each muscle: the insertional activity, fibrillations, positive sharp waves, and recruitment patterns. Space is necessary for describing motor unit potentials by form, amplitude, duration, and frequencies. About one-third of the work sheet should be reserved for comments and an impression.

Information about the nerve conduction test may also be included on this form. The form should be simply designed for ease of reading but yet inclusive of pertinent data. One sheet is usually sufficient for recording the entire electrophysiologic examination. The form must always be signed at the bottom by the examiner.

SUMMARY

Electromyography is the study of the electrical activity of muscle. In diseases affecting the motor unit, abnormal electrical activity may be detected and studied.

Electromyographic studies are of considerable value to the physician in clarifying the neuromuscular and musculoskeletal status of some patients. The EMG needle examination is one approach to providing this information.

The electromyographer is an individual who combines his knowledge of anatomy, physiology, neuromuscular pathology, instrumentation, and the clinical aspects of neuromuscular and musculoskeletal diseases to assess the patient. He uses electrophysiologic methods to study the electrical activity of muscle. The electromyographer, by providing valuable information, assists the physician who can then make a diagnosis.

The successful use of electromyography in medicine requires, in addition to knowledge of the subject areas mentioned, experience. This experience is best gained by serving an apprenticeship with an experienced electromyographer and by many electromyographic examinations.

The discussion here is introductory and should provide a starting point for the reader who wants to understand electromyography (needle examination) as a clarifying tool.

REFERENCES

1. Lambert EH: Electromyography and electric stimulation of peripheral nerves and muscle. In: Clinical Examinations in Neurology, Mayo Clinic and Mayo Foundation. Philadelphia, WB Saunders, 1976
2. Adrian ED, Bronk DW: The discharge of impulses in motor nerve fibers. J Physiol 67: 119–151, 1929
3. Weddell G, Feinstein B, Pattle RE: The electrical activity of voluntary muscle in man under normal and pathological conditions. Brain 67:178–257, 1944
4. Cohen HL, Brumlik J: Manual of Electroneuromyography, 2nd edn. New York, Harper and Row, 1977
5. Goodgold J, Eberstein A: Electrodiagnosis of Neuromuscular Diseases, 2nd edn. Baltimore, Williams and Wilkins, 1978
6. Kraft GH: Peripheral Neuropathies. In: Practical Electromyography, ed. Johnson EW. Baltimore, Williams and Wilkins, 1980
7. Lenman JAR, Ritchie AE: Clinical Electromyography, 2nd edn. New York, JB Lippincott, 1977
8. Smorto MP, Basmajian JV: Electrodiagnosis: A Handbook for Neurologists. New York, Harper and Row, 1977
9. Feinstein B, Lindegard B, Nyman E, et al: Morphologic studies of motor units in normal muscles. Acta Anat 23: 127–142, 1955
10. Edstrom L, Kugelberg E: Histochemical composition, distribution of fibers and fatigability of single motor units. J Neurol Neurosurg Psychiatry 31: 424–433, 1968
11. Buchthal F, Guld C, Rosenfalck P: Multielectrode study of the territory of a motor unit. Acta Physiol Scand 39: 83–104, 1957
12. Coërs C, Woolf AL: The Innervation of Muscle: A Biopsy Study. Springfield, Thomas, 1959
13. Elmqvist D: Neuromuscular transmission defects. In: Electrodiagnosis and Electromyography, 3rd edn., ed. Licht S. Baltimore, Waverly Press, 1971
14. Guld D, Rosenfalck A, Willison RG: Report of committee on EMG instrumentation. Electroencephalogr Clin Neurophysiol 28:399–413, 1970

15. Karselis T: Descriptive Medical Electronics and Instrumentation. Thorofare, NJ, Charles Slack, 1973
16. Mulder DW, Rosenbaum RA, Layton DD: Late progression of poliomyelitis or forme fruste amyotrophic lateral sclerosis. Mayo Clinic Proc 47:756–761, 1972
17. Dyken MC, Smith OM, Peake RC: An electromyographic diagnostic screening test in McArdle's disease and case report. Neurology 17: 45–50, 1967

4 | The Use of Conduction Velocity Measurements as an Evaluative Tool

John L. Echternach

INTRODUCTION TO NERVE CONDUCTION

Once it was understood that in human physiology there is a relationship between peripheral nerves and reactions to stimuli, interest was focused on how rapidly this information could be conducted to the nervous system as a reaction occurred. Some of the very earliest attempts to measure nerve conduction velocity were based on mental processes. Even though the assumptions on which these attempts were based were erroneous, some of the early estimates of nerve conduction velocity were remarkably accurate. More sophisticated estimates of nerve conduction velocity were attempted by Von Helmholtz in the mid 1800s. Using electrical stimuli to cause muscle contraction and improved devices for measuring time, he undertook a series of experiments in which he is reported to have measured conduction velocity in the median nerve.[1, 2]

As technology advanced, more adequate methods of measuring nerve conduction which could be used with fairly good accuracy in the laboratory were developed. However, the clinical usefulness of these measurements was not recognized until 1948 when Hodes, Larrabee, and German published their study on the conduction velocity of the median nerve of the upper extremity.[3] They stimulated the median nerve at the elbow and at the wrist, recording the reaction of the abductor pollicis brevis muscle of the hand to each stimulus. The time required for the impulse to travel from the wrist to the hand muscle was subtracted from the time required for the impulse to travel from the elbow to the same hand muscle and the difference used to calculate a conduction time over a nerve segment by measuring, on the skin, the distance between the wrist and the elbow. They then calculated a conduction velocity by taking this remaining time interval and dividing it into the distance on the skin. This velocity, in a motor nerve, was expressed in meters per second (m/s).

Since this first published report, clinical conduction velocity measurements have been of great interest as a diagnostic tool. Literally hundreds of publications have reported normal motor nerve conduction velocity of the easily excessible motor nerves of the upper and lower extremities as well as abnormal findings in a great variety of pathologic conditions.

Later, as equipment and techniques improved, sensory nerve conduction velocity was also studied. These measurements have been widely applied clinically to investigate specific neuropathic processes as well as compression syndromes in both the upper and lower extremity. Nerve conduction velocity measurements are frequently combined with electromyographic studies to obtain a more complete physiologic picture of the patient's problem.

The combination of electromyographic and nerve conduction velocity studies has been termed *electroneuromyography.* Clinically, motor and sensory nerve conduction velocities are often measured prior to electromyographic studies. The advantage to this routine is that in many instances nerve conduction studies, by themselves, provide the answer to a clinical problem. When they do not, their combination with electromyographic studies gives a much better picture of the pathology.

Clinical nerve conduction studies can best be understood by looking at the basic process of conduction in a single neuron and then applying this information to clinical nerve conduction studies. If a single neuron receives an adequate stimulus, then electrical activity is conducted from the cell body along its peripheral axon. The rate at which this electrical impulse is conducted to its synapse is essentially the measurement of conduction velocity. There are two important physiologic concepts to be aware of when conduction velocity studies are being considered.[4]

The more highly myelinated the axon is, the more rapidly it will conduct impulses. The type of conduction that takes place in peripheral axons is called saltatory, since the myelin sheath of peripheral axons is discontinuous. Conduction precedes from one node of Ranvier to the next in a jumping fashion, increasing the velocity along the course of the myelinated nerve. Once the electrical impulse reaches the end of the axon and is at the synapse, an entirely new process begins. Nerve conduction measurements along the course of the axon are not involved with the time it takes to cross a synapse, or, in the case of motor nerves, the time it would take to cross the motor endplate.

In the clinical situation stimulation to the peripheral nerve will activate thousands of axons. The resulting response is the recording of a compound muscle action potential (Fig. 4-1). The *conduction time* or *latency* is the time from the point where the electrical stimulation is applied until the muscle begins to contract. This time represents the conduction of the fastest fibers in the mixed peripheral nerve. By stimulating over a peripheral nerve at two sites, a conduction velocity can be

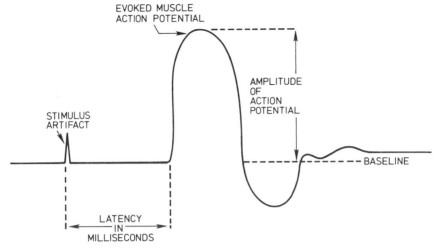

Fig. 4-1.   Elements of the evoked muscle action potential.

determined between them. Conduction time over the course of the nerve can be determined by subtracting the latency of the distal site from that of the proximal site (Fig. 4-2). The difference is divided into the distance measured on the surface between the two stimulation sites and over the course of the peripheral nerve. In this way a gross but reasonably adequate estimate of nerve conduction velocity can be obtained.

Sensory nerve conduction velocity studies follow the same principle as those of motor conduction velocity studies, with one major difference.[5, 6] In sensory conduction, stimulation is over the course of the nerve and recording is also from the nerve. There is no intervening motor endplate or other structure. Sensory studies may be done in one of two ways: the orthodromic method involves stimulating over a sensory area and recording from the nerve in a proximal region, thus duplicating the process that occurs in the normal situation with sensory information being gathered in the periphery and carried proximally by the sensory fibers.

Sensory nerves may also be studied by providing antidromic simulation. The recording is in a primary sensory area, but stimulation occurs at the mixed nerve. Velocities are calculated in the same manner as for motor nerves, stimulating proximal and distal sites and subtracting the distal site from the proximal site. Theoretically, sensory conduction velocities can be computed for the distal segment alone as long as allowances are made for the fact that between the recording electrode and the sensory nerve there are intervening soft tissues, which will distort the values of the computed conduction velocity making them appear to be slower than they really are.

When clinical conduction velocity studies are done, the interpretation is not of velocities alone, but includes several other factors. Factors that may be interpreted in a conduction velocity study are: (1) conduction time or latency, (2) amplitude of response, (3) waveform, and (4) velocities.

The *conduction time* or *latency* from each stimulation site is particularly im-

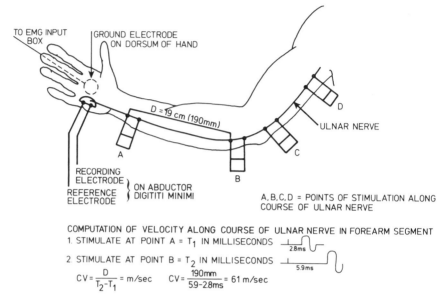

Fig. 4-2. An example of nerve conduction velocity computation. The ulnar nerve is stimulated at the sites illustrated and velocities between sites of stimulation calculated.

portant for the distal site of stimulation, since no velocity can be computed for this segment in motor studies. Comparisons of distal latency with normals reported in studies or with a comparable area in the same individual over a normal segment yields valuable information. An example of this would be stimulation of the median nerve at the wrist, above the carpal tunnel, when a compression lesion is suspected at the carpal tunnel. This lesion is between the site of stimulation and the recording electrodes on the abductor pollicis brevis. Latency provides the most critical information about the median nerve, which, if compressed at the wrist, will be prolonged.

In many conditions, and particularly in compression lesions, the *amplitude* of the *recorded action potential* is decreased when stimulating above the site of compression. The amplitude of response must be compared with sites stimulated above and below the site of compression. Also, in many conditions, the number of conducting axons is decreased. Therefore, the amplitude of the response may be diminished, compared to that of other normal nerves in the same individual.

When stimulating several sites over the same nerve, it is very important that the *shape of the action potential* stay nearly the same to assure that the same nerve is being stimulated. Secondly, the action potential is often distorted, depending on the disease process affecting the nerve. There is some research evidence indicating that the rate at which the action potential reaches its maximum peak may be an important factor in the interpretation of action potentials.

Lastly, the factor interpreted and reported most commonly in the literature is a change in conduction velocity. Ordinarily, reported *changes in conduction speed* are considered abnormal if velocity is slowed. Conduction velocity abnormalities may be confined to a particular nerve segment (as in compression lesions), along the entire course of the nerve (as in Charcot-Marie-Tooth disease), or over the distal segment of nerve. The locus for slowing depends on the disease process under investigation. Normative conduction velocity values provided by Sunderland[7] are important for clinicians. Many investigators have suggested that each laboratory develop its own set of normal values based on technique and instrumentation.

INSTRUMENTATION

[handwritten annotation: $Hz = 1-2$ output $= 0-250$ V]

The instrumentation used in performing nerve conduction velocity has two major components. The first is a stimulator to excite the nerve with electrical current and the second is an amplifier system to record the results of this stimulation.

Modern electromyographic equipment includes a stimulator capable of delivering a rectangular pulse, the duration of which can vary from .05 to .2 ms. The interval between pulses is variable, but is controlled by the clinician. Most examiners stimulate at a frequency of 1 or 2 pulses per second. Most units provide a wider range of available frequencies so that other evoked potential studies may be performed using the stimulator. The output of the stimulator should allow a supramaximal stimulus to activate an entire peripheral nerve. The intensity of current should vary from 0 to approximately 250 V. The stimulus is delivered to the nerve through bipolar electrodes separated by 2.5 to 3 cm. The diameter of the electrodes should be about 1 cm. Most stimulators provide an additional set of jacks so that ring electrodes or flexible paired electrodes may be used in place of bipolar electrodes with fixed interelectrode separation.

The recording system includes a set of recording electrodes which are applied to the patient. For motor conduction studies, these electrodes are usually paired and flexible, having silver-silver chloride recording discs each 1 cm in diameter. For sensory conduction, a variety of electrodes have been used for stimulating over sensory fibers. An example is the flexible ring electrode, which can be secured tightly around a finger. The response obtained at these recording electrodes are then led into a preamplifier to magnify or enlarge the muscle action potential or the sensory potential. This is the first stage of amplification. The next step is a second stage of amplification and display of the activity.

The most common display unit is an oscilloscope where each sweep of the oscilloscope is triggered by the stimulus. The oscilloscope displays a stimulus deflection (artifact) followed by a deflection caused by the action potential. Advances in electronics have permitted this display to be stored in a variety of ways, including the use of phosphors to retain the image until it is erased electronically or a digital storage system can be used in which the oscilloscope sweep is analyzed and redisplayed. This storage capability allows the examiner to observe the recorded phenomenon at leisure and to make certain measurements of the wave while it is stored.

Permanent records of the oscilloscope display range from a polaroid picture to a fiber optic recording system that duplicates exactly what is seen on the oscilloscope screen. Also, forms of paper recording have been utilized in some equipment. An additional feature of most electromyographic units is the ability to simultaneously present the information on a loudspeaker. This can be done during nerve conduction velocity testing. During nerve stimulation the sound of the response can often give the examiner a clue as to whether he is close to or on the nerve trunk. The more crisp and sharp the sound of the action potential, the more likely the nerve is being stimulated directly.

Additional devices have been designed for easier nerve conduction velocity testing. The first of these measures latencies or conduction time directly. This device allows oscilloscopic measurements from the stimulus artifact to the displayed action potential and also provides a direct readout in milliseconds of this latency or conduction time. This device is commonly called a strobe or a latency indicator. Another very useful device for conduction velocity studies, especially sensory studies, is a signal averager. An averager takes a preselected number of stimuli, averages their output, and displays one trace that is an average of the several stimuli. This method discriminates against random noise and displays a "clean" action potential that makes measurement and analysis easier, especially when the size of the response is quite small (a few microvolts).

To summarize, a stimulator is required to deliver the electrical stimulus to the nerve. A recording system is then needed to record the resulting action potential. This recording method usually involves two processes: (1) an instant display telling the examiner that the desired information is obtained and (2) a method for permanently recording the results for more leisurely analyzing and documenting the record.

BASIC TESTING PROCEDURES FOR THE NERVES IN THE UPPER EXTREMITIES

Median and Ulnar Nerve Conduction Procedures

The muscle selected for recording motor responses to median nerve conduction testing is the abductor pollicis brevis.[8-10] This muscle is easily found, but before the electrodes are applied in any motor nerve procedure, the skin should be prepared. A simple, but basic routine that can be adopted is the following: sandpaper the area lightly with very fine sandpaper; clean the area with alcohol; then dry the area by rubbing it vigorously with gauze. This procedure assures that skin oils and accumulated dead skin are removed and provides a uniform method for skin preparation for motor nerve conduction testing. The recording electrode should be placed in approximately the center of the muscle belly over the motor endplate area. The reference electrode should be placed a minimum of 2.5 to 3 cm distally and can be placed over the flexor tendon area of thumb. Electrodes should be securely attached to prevent movement during the course of stimulation. The median nerve can then be stimulated.

The distal point of stimulation is at the wrist. Since the carpal tunnel is often a site of involvement in the median nerve, this point of stimulation should be above the flexor retinaculum. A reliable method for determining the course of the median nerve at the wrist is to find the flexor carpi radialis and palmaris longus tendons. The median nerve can be found between these two tendons. A suggested method is to measure 10 cm from the recording electrode over the abductor pollicis brevis muscle and to stimulate at this point.

The next site of stimulation of the median nerve is at the elbow, just medial to the biceps tendon as the nerve descends into the forearm and crosses the medial epicondyle. Above the elbow, the median nerve can be stimulated anywhere proximal to the medial epicondyle, along the medial aspect of the humerus all the way to the axilla. The ulnar and median nerves run parallel to each other at this location so stimulation should be given lateral to the ulnar nerve. If this procedure is followed, the muscle action potential does not change in shape with increasing stimulation.

The third site of stimulation can be in the mid to upper arm or the axilla. Stimulation at these points gives a reasonably long segment above the elbow so that conduction velocity can be calculated for the upper arm segment as well as for a segment from the elbow to the wrist. The median nerve can be involved in compression problems in the axilla, so sometimes it is important to stimulate the median nerve in the supraclavicular area at the posterior cervical triangle above the clavicle. Stimulation here is over the brachial plexus, not over the median nerve directly so that a conduction velocity in the segment from the supraclavicular area to the axilla or upper arm can be calculated.

The method just described permits evaluation of the median nerve in segments from: (1) the supraclavicular region to the upper arm, (2) from the upper arm to the elbow, and (3) from the elbow to the wrist. It also permits an interpretation of the latency from stimulating at the wrist to the recording electrode on the abductor pollis brevis. Occasionally the anterior interosseous branch of the median nerve, which innervates the flexor pollicis longus distally, is involved.[11-14] This involvement occurs sometimes by trauma or by a compression syndrome in this area. A variation in technique is required when involvement of this nerve is suspected. Recording electrodes must be placed over the flexor pollicis longus and the subject stimulated at the elbow. Recording for both the flexor pollicis longus and the abductor pollicis brevis will determine whether this branch of the nerve is involved because conduction to the abductor pollicis brevis will remain normal but conduction time or latency to the flexor pollicis longus will either be absent or abnormally long.

In performing median nerve motor conduction velocity tests the subject's arm should be comfortably placed at his side and the palm supinated. Measurements on the skin are taken in the same position in which the patient was stimulated. A caliper should be used for measurements from the supraclavicular region to the axilla or upper arm because measuring over the contour of the body with a tape measure tends to distort the distance. All other measurements may be done adequately with a tape measure or caliper. For consistent measurements, the same technique should be used all the time.

Ulnar motor nerve conduction determinations are very similar to those done on the median nerve except for two important differences:[8] the first is that positioning of the upper extremity for the ulnar nerve is best done with the elbow flexed to 90° and the shoulder abducted to 90° and externally rotated.[15] This places the ulnar nerve in a position, at the elbow, which represents its true length. The recording electrode is placed at the motor point over the abductor digiti minimi, and the reference electrode is placed 3 cm or more away over the flexor tendon to the fifth finger. Stimulation of the ulnar nerve is then carried out at the wrist, approximately 10 cm from the recording electrode and just lateral to the flexor carpi ulnaris tendon.

The next two points of stimulation are above and below the elbow. A segment of nerve across the elbow must be examined since pathology of the ulna at the elbow is so common.[16-18] The site below the elbow is found just before the nerve becomes deep, entering the flexor carpi ulnaris after crossing the ulnar groove at the elbow. The site above the elbow should be a minimum of 10 cm proximal to the previous site. Shorter segments tend to maximize error measurements.

The next site of stimulation of the ulnar nerve is high in the medial upper arm or in the axilla. The ulnar nerve parallels the median nerve in the area of the inner arm area and the nerve can can be stimulated along its entire course. The ulnar nerve can also be stimulated at the brachial plexus in the supraclavicular region, as described earlier for the median nerve. Using this site of stimulation, conduction velocities for the ulnar nerve can be calculated in: (1) the segment from the supraclavicular region to the axilla or upper arm; (2) from the axilla or upper arm area to the site above the elbow; (3) from above the elbow to below the elbow; and (4) from below the elbow to the wrist. Also a latency can be obtained from the wrist to the abductor digiti minimi.

A useful variation on the ulnar nerve motor conduction measurement is necessary when involvement of the deep branch to the hand is suspected.[19-21] A second site in the hand should be selected for recording. The site most commonly used is the first dorsal interosseous muscle. Surface electrodes are placed over this muscle, the nerve is stimulated as before at the wrist, and a latency to the first dorsal interosseous is recorded. This latency is then compared with that obtained at the abductor. If the difference is such that the latency to the first dorsal interosseous is more than 1.5 ms longer than that to the abductor digiti minimi, pathology in the deep branch of the ulnar nerve may be implicated.

Normal latency for the ulnar and median nerves, when stimulated at the wrist using a 10-cm segment, should be less than 4 ms. It is a good practice, when examining for pathology in the ulnar or median nerve, to always include the other nerve in the examination to provide a comparison. Some investigators feel that it is more valid to compare the distal latency of the ulnar and median nerve in the same extremity rather than compare the nerves in opposite extremities. In determining whether there is slowing of the distal latency, a difference of more than 1 ms on comparison is considered abnormal. This is a more sensitive indicator than a cut-off of 4 ms. Obviously when a large number of individuals are examined, here is a great deal of variation in forearm and hand sizes. For this reason, the distance from the point of stimulation to the pick-up electrode should be standardized to improve the possibility of comparisons in this distal segment.

Conduction velocity of the forearm segment in both the ulnar and median nerves is usually slightly slower than the upper arm segment. This observation is typical of peripheral nerves in general. A possible reason for this phenomenon is that the distal segments are cooler and therefore conduct more slowly.[22, 23] A normal conduction velocity value for the median nerve from the elbow to the wrist is 55 m/s; from axilla or upper arm to the elbow, 65 m/s; and from the supraclavicular site to the upper arm, 65 to 70 m/s. On the ulnar nerve, the forearm segment usually conducts at approximately 55 m/s; across the elbow at 45 to 50 m/s; in the upper arm at 60 to 65 m/s; and from the supraclavicular site to the axilla at 65 to 70 m/s. Slowing across the elbow segment occurs if the nerve conducts 10 m/s more slowly than the segment below it, or 20 m/s slower than the segment above it. The ulnar nerve normally conducts more slowly across the elbow than the segments above and below it, because it is cooled at this superficial location.[8, 15]

Radial Motor Nerve Conduction
Procedure

The radial nerve was the last motor nerve of the upper extremity to be studied using motor nerve conduction techniques. This nerve is technically more difficult to study than the ulnar and median nerves because areas where the nerve may be stimulated are not as readily accessible. The technique used most commonly today evolved over the course of time and was developed by several authors.[25, 26-30]

Because of surface measurement problems at the proximal location of the nerve and of proper electrode placement, valid recordings are difficult to obtain. Currently, the most commonly used technique is to apply surface electrodes over the extensor pollicis longus in the forearm, with the active electrode over the belly of the muscle and the reference electrode in the area of the radial styloid. The most common sites of stimulation are: the forearm, approximately 6 to 10 cm above the recording electrode; the elbow, in the area of the brachioradialis and at the lateral arm as the radial nerve descends in the intermuscular septum between the biceps and triceps muscles approximately 10 cm above the lateral epicondyle. The nerve can also be stimulated in the midaxilla and in the area above the clavicle. Recent studies have indicated that estimating velocities from the supraclavicular area to the axilla is unreliable and that perhaps axillary stimulation should not be attempted unless it is specifically justified.[31] Segmental velocities are usually calculated for the area from the supraclavicular region to the lateral arm and from the lateral arm to the forearm. Normal conduction velocity for these two segments are 65 to 70 m/s for the upper segment of the nerve and 55 to 65 m/s for the lower segment of the nerve. The wave form of the recorded muscle action potential to stimulation of the radial nerve often shows a small but consistently present positive deflection when stimulating at the forearm and elbow sites but less often present in the upper arm area and supraclavicular sites.[30] This finding presents difficulties in determining latency because of differences in initial deflection between the lower and upper portions of the nerves.

Sensory Nerve Conduction Studies—Median and Ulnar Nerves. Sensory nerve conductions are performed routinely on the ulnar and median nerve and frequently on the radial nerve.[10, 28, 32, 33, 36] There are two commonly employed techniques for sensory conduction velocity studies of the median and ulnar nerves. The orthodromic technique to the median nerve involves stimulation through digital ring electrodes applied over the second digit with the sensory action potential recorded over the mixed median nerve at the wrist, elbow, or upper arm sites. In this method, the motor nerve stimulation sites become recording sites for the sensory conduction study. An antidromic technique can also be used. With this technique, recordings are made from digital electrodes over the second digit with the nerve stimulated at the wrist, elbow, and upper arm sites (that is, the same as in conducting a motor nerve study). In studies comparing the results of orthodromic and antidromic stimulation, there is no statistically significant difference in the latencies on velocities obtained. However, the amplitude of sensory potentials is larger with the antidromic technique. The major disadvantage of the antidromic technique stems from movement artifact following stimulation of a mixed nerve. The artifact may obscure a very small sensory potential.

The technique for evoking ulnar nerve sensory conduction velocities is very similar. Digital ring electrodes are applied over the fifth finger. Either this site is stimulated through the digital nerve while recording over the mixed nerve, or the digital electrodes become recording sites and the stimulation is applied over the mixed nerve in the same sites as used for motor nerve conduction testing. Often in the clinical situation the only sensory testing done is by stimulating at the distal site and recording through the digits. In this case the major factors examined are distal latency and amplitude of response. In normal individuals, using modern equipment it is not uncommon to obtain 30 to 50 μV responses in both the ulnar and medial nerves. The amplitude of response diminishes with aging, and this becomes noticeable in individuals 60 years of age and older.

Radial Sensory Nerve Conduction

Sensory conduction testing is most valuable when it is combined with motor nerve testing and is rarely done alone. Sensory conduction velocity techniques for the radial nerve involved palpation to find the distal branches of the superficial radial nerve as they cross the radial aspect of the styloid process or as they cross the extensor tendons.[28, 33, 34] Recording electrodes are then placed in this area with the recording electrode being proximal and the reference electrode being distal. Stimulation is applied approximately 10 to 14 cm above the recording electrodes in the forearm where the superficial radial nerve accompanies the cephalic vein. Other sites of stimulation on the radial nerve are at the elbow or lateral arm site, and velocities can be calculated for these segments.

The response amplitude using this antidromic technique is often 40 to 50 μV.

Sensory nerve testing may help to localize a radial nerve lesion by considering the site at which the superficial radial nerve divides from the main branch.

Other Nerves in the Upper Extremity

Other motor nerves in the upper extremities, which can also be tested, include the musculocutaneous and axillary nerves.[38-42] Nelson and Currier[38] reported a method for studying the musculocutaneous nerve, which included applying electrodes to the biceps brachii and then stimulating the musculocutaneous nerve at the axilla and in the posterior triangle of the neck above the clavicle. They reported a mean value of 74 m/s with a range of 60 to 89 m/s.

The method for stimulating the axillary nerve is very similar. The recording electrodes are placed over the deltoid muscle and the nerve is stimulated above the clavicle in the posterior triangle and in the posterior axilla.[42] Reported velocities are generally between 65 to 75 m/s. Gassel and Kraft[43, 41] have studied the brachial plexus extensively and have reported latencies to shoulder girdle muscles, including the supraspinatus, infraspinatus, and serratus anterior, as a method for studying lesions in this area. A method for studying sensory conduction in the musculocutaneous nerve has been reported by Trojaborg,[40] and by Spindler and Felsenthal.[44]

BASIC TESTING PROCEDURES FOR NERVES IN THE LOWER EXTREMITY—MOTOR CONDUCTION TECHNIQUES

The motor nerves commonly tested in the lower extremity are: the tibial, peroneal, and femoral.[9, 45-49] The tibial and peroneal nerve techniques were developed earlier than that for the femoral nerve, most likely because of the much greater incidence of tibial and peroneal nerve pathologies.

Tibial Nerve

The technique for examining the motor portion of the tibial nerve is as follows: the recording electrode is usually placed over the belly of the abductor hallucis muscle and the reference electrode is placed 3 to 5 cm distally. The ground electrode may be placed over the dorsum of the foot or over the lateral malleolus.

Points of stimulation for the tibial nerve are behind the medial malleolus and in the mid popliteal space. To improve accuracy and patient comfort, it is best to test the patient in the prone position with the knee slightly flexed and a roll under the ankle. This procedure reduces tension over the popiteal space so that pressure can be applied on the stimulating electrodes at this site.

This method tests the motor portion of the tibial nerve through the medial planter nerve branch. If a lesion is suspected in the lateral planter nerve, then recording can be done from the abductor digiti minimi muscle of the fifth toe. The stimulation sites would remain the same. Stimulation at the medial malleolus, should be at a point above the flexor retinaculum, especially when a compression causing a tarsal tunnel syndrome, is suspected.[50–54]

Peroneal Nerve

For motor conduction studies of the peroneal nerve, a recording electrode is placed over the extensor digitorum brevis. The reference electrode is placed distally over the dorsum of the foot or over the tendon of the fifth toe. The ground electrode should be between the recording and reference electrodes.

Points of stimulation on the peroneal nerve are: the anterior ankle just lateral to the tibialis anterior tendon and slightly above the level of the malleoli; just below the head of the fibula; and the lateral aspect of the popliteal space. These sites include two segments to measure conduction on the peroneal nerve. One segment crossing the fibular head is a common site of peroneal nerve compression. A second segment from below the fibular head to the anterior ankle should be examined.[53, 54]

To test the peroneal nerve the patient should be placed in a supine position with the knee slightly flexed and supported on a roll or pillow. When the peroneal and tibial nerves in the lower extremity are tested, the most distal portion of the sciatic nerve is actually being examined. A technique for conduction velocity measurement of the sciatic nerve itself has been reported.[55] This technique is difficult and requires stimulation applied through needle electrodes, which are inserted just below the gluteal cleft and close to the sciatic nerve. Recording is then done at the popliteal space directly from the tibial and peroneal nerves.

Femoral Nerve

Gassel first used femoral nerve conduction techniques by stimulating the femoral nerve in the femoral triangle and recording from the quadriceps at different intervals. The conduction velocity was computed between the recording sites on the quadriceps.[47] Echternach and Hayden reported a method of stimulating the femoral triangle and the adductor canal (Hunter's canal).[48] The recording electrode was placed over the vastus medialis, the reference electrode over the femoral condyle, and the ground electrode over the upper tibial shaft.

Johnson[49] reported a similar method but added a stimulation site above the inquinal ligament, allowing velocity on the femoral nerve to be computed from two segments: one crossing the inquinal ligament region, and a distal segment in the thigh. This technique allows one to compute a velocity across a common site of entrapment of the femoral nerve.[49]

Normal conduction velocity of the peroneal nerve is usually in the range of 45 to 60 m/s, with any value below 40 m/s considered as abnormally slowed. The same is true for the tibial nerve. Reported velocities for the femoral nerve are in the 65 to 70 m/s range, with velocities below 55 m/s considered as abnormally slow conduction.

Sensory Nerve Conduction Techniques in the Lower Extremity. Sensory nerve conduction techniques in the lower extremity have been known for many years,[56, 57] but due to averaging techniques, they have been performed clinically with increasing frequency during the past 10 years. Microvoltages in lower extremity sensory nerves among patients with abnormalities may be extremely small. Averaging of these abnormal potentials is essential if they are to be detected. The sural is the most commonly tested lower extremity sensory nerve.[58-63] The most common technique for conduction velocity testing on the sural nerve is .5–.75 inches below the lateral malleolus parallel to a line drawn through the tip of the lateral malleolus. These electrodes are 3 cm apart. Good skin preparation is essential. Stimulation is given 14 to 17 cm above the recording electrode over the lateral aspect of the calf. The sural nerve runs just anterior to the achilles tendon and is easily found for stimulation. The ground electrode should be placed between the stimulating and recording electrode over the medial malleous. Amplitudes of the sural nerve action potential recorded in this fashion are normally 30 to 50 μV. The latency reported on the sural nerve for a 14-cm segment is 3.5 ms.[59]

FACIAL NERVE—MOTOR CONDUCTION VELOCITY DETERMINATION

A motor nerve latency can be obtained by stimulating the facial nerve below the ear and anterior to the mastoid process and recording the conduction time to a muscle on the face. The first studies were reported by Brown,[64] who used the mentalis muscle for recording his response. He reported normal latencies of 3.5 to 4.3 ms. Several authors have also reported latency values in various muscles of the face, including the orbicularis oris and frontalis.[65-68] Johnson reported a mean latency value of 4 ms, with a range of 3 to 5 ms. The placement of the ground electrode when the facial nerve is to be stimulated is very important because the stimulus artifact will sometimes be so large that interpretation of the deflection of the muscle action potential waveform is difficult and accurate computation of conduction time may be a problem.[66, 67] This problem can sometimes be corrected by repositioning the ground electrode. Several authors have placed a ground electrode over the angle of the mandible, while others have used a small EEG needle in the scalp as a ground electrode.[57] The most common condition in which the facial nerve is evaluated is idiopathic Bells palsy; other causes of facial weakness include trauma and diabetes mellitus.[67, 69]

CLINICAL VALUE OF NERVE CONDUCTION STUDIES

Nerve conduction tests are a very important aspect of the evaluation of lower motor neuron disorders and represent the most reliable method for testing the functional status of a nerve. Combining this form of testing with electromyography often provides a more complete understanding of the patient's problems than either of these tests alone. The literature on nerve conduction velocity testing has become extensive, and the procedure is applicable to many neuromuscular conditions.

When considering the performance of nerve conduction velocity testing, certain basic ideas must be kept in mind. The first is that testing of any kind is never performed without a complete and thorough understanding of the patient's problem from his history and from clinical examination. The history, clinical examination, and assessment of clinical findings are essential for planning the electrophysiology evaluation. Secondly, when planning a nerve conduction velocity measurement, testing of only one nerve will be inadequate. Even with clearly defined problems, a minimum of two nerves in any one extremity should be examined. Testing should be continued until the examiner is convinced that a normal area cannot be found.

Conduction studies have basically been used to demonstrate whether conduction along the course of the nerve is normal, abnormal, or absent. One major use of conduction studies has been to localize compressive lesions. Conduction studies also have been done to demonstrate whether conduction is normal in the presence of myopathic disease; that is, some parameters of the conduction study are abnormal but conduction velocity remains normal. Nerve conduction studies may assist in localizing a lesion. Sometimes conduction velocities are used to demonstrate that only motor or sensory fibers are involved, as in ALS or motor neuron disease in which there is no sensory component.

ENTRAPMENT AND COMPRESSION SYNDROMES

This section briefly addresses the major entrapment and compression syndromes for which conduction velocity testing has made a positive contribution to the understanding and evaluation of the problem.

Carpal Tunnel Syndrome

This condition is characterized by entrapment of the median nerve under the flexor retinaculum at the carpal tunnel. In most instances, the patient's first complaint is a tingling, burning or numbness in the sensory distribution supplied by the median nerve in the hand. The patient's problem is usually worse at night but is improved by shaking or rubbing the hands. Entrapment has been suggested as the most common cause of upper extremity pain.[70] On evaluation, patients may show atrophy and weakness of the thenar eminence. Often they will show changes in sensory distribution of the median nerve to the hand, such as decreased sensation to touch or pin prick. Many patients will have a positive Phalen sign (an increase in their sensory complaints when the wrist is held in full flexion or full extension). The multitude of causes for carpal tunnel syndrome include: trauma, pregnancy, local tumors or other growths in the carpal tunnel, hypothyroidism,[71-73] or anatomic variations of the content of the carpal tunnel.[74] Nerve conduction studies will reveal prolonged distal latencies of motor and/or sensory fibers of the medial nerve.[73, 75] On comparison with the ulnar nerve in the same extremity, there is usually more than a 1-ms difference over a similar segment of the nerve. Depending on the severity of compression, the amplitude of the motor or sensory response may be reduced.[75]

Ulnar Nerve Entrapment

Common sites of compression or entrapment on the ulnar nerve are at the elbow and the tunnel of Guyon at the wrist.[17–21] Entrapment of the nerve at the cupital tunnel has many causes, the most common of which is recurrent or single severe trauma around the elbow.[10, 70] Generally, patients complain of numbness, or paresthesia in the ulnar nerve distribution with increased symptoms on percussion over the nerve. Prolonged elbow flexion or leaning on the elbow also evoke complaints. The usual conduction velocity finding is slowing in the segment across the elbow. The below-elbow stimulation site should be as distal as possible to be sure that the lesion is included within the above-to-below elbow segment. Compressive lesions of the ulnar nerve at the wrist are in the tunnel of Guyon in which the nerve passes between the pisiform bone and the hook of the hamate. Motor branches arise with the canal to the hypothenar eminence, and the deep branch begins as the nerve exits the canal.[74] At this location, sometimes there is sparing of the innervation to the abductor digital minimi with only the deep branch of the ulnar nerve being involved. In patients with suspected entrapment of the ulnar nerve at the wrist or elbow, sensory conduction testing should also be included. Sensory testing will often show a decrease in response amplitude and greater abnormalities than revealed by the motor conduction tests.

Thoracic Outlet Syndromes

Another site of upper extremity nerve compression involves symptoms that may be similar to those of ulnar nerve compression caused by thoracic outlet syndromes.[76–79] When compression takes place at the junction of the scalenus muscles and the first rib, parasthesia is often present in the ulnar aspect of the arm and hand. If the lesion is severe, ulnar motor conduction velocity may be reduced. The most likely finding is reduced sensory amplitudes of the ulnar nerve. The involvement is usually at the lower trunk of the brachial plexus with thinning or compression at the site of the first rib and insertion of the scalenus anterior muscle. For this type of suspected thoracic outlet syndrome all segments of the ulnar nerve should be tested. The site of stimulation in the supraclavicular area, however, is usually below the site of the lesion and it is unlikely that segmental slowing of ulnar motor conduction velocity can be demonstrated.

Radial Nerve Compression

Compression of the radial nerve is most common at the site where the nerve emerges from the intramuscular septum. The triceps muscle is usually spared, with symptoms involving the wrist and finger extensors.[80]

The posterior interosseous nerve is the continuation of the radial nerve that descends along the posterior interosseous membrane after it has given off motor branches to the brachioradialis and extensor carpi radialis longus and brevis. This nerve may be compressed as it passes through the supinator muscle. The patient complains of difficulty when extending the thumb and fingers; but the wrist extensors are intact and no sensory loss is present.[82] Nerve conduction studies are directed at showing slowing in the segment between sites of stimulation in the lateral arm and the forearm.[83] Sometimes it is difficult to demonstrate much change in radial nerve conduction in this condition and EMG will help to clarify the problem. The radial nerve can also be involved in its upper portion by pressure from fractures about the radial spiral groove.[84] When these problems are encountered, it is important to demonstrate the higher level of the lesion along the course of the nerve and to determine the severity of compression.

Peroneal Nerve Entrapment

The most common compressive lesion of the peroneal nerve occurs at the fibular head. Nerve conduction velocity studies should be directed at demonstrating slowing in the segment across the fibular head by computing and comparing a velocity for this segment and the segment below it. The major clinical finding in peroneal palsy is a foot drop or dorsiflexion weakness. The most common mechanism of peroneal nerve compression is sitting in a cross-legged position for prolonged periods of time.[53] Other reasons for compression of the peroneal nerve as it crosses the fibular head include direct trauma, pressure of a cast, limb positioning or compression during surgical procedures.[54, 85]

Tibial Nerve Entrapment

The most common compression injury is at the tarsal tunnel, posterior and inferior to the medial malleolus, where the nerve is covered by the flexor retinaculum. Accompanying the tibial nerve in the tarsal tunnel are tendons and major blood vessels. Abnormal findings within the tarsal tunnel or due to a variety of other causes have been described[50-52] and may be associated with foot deformities and prolonged weakness of the lower leg and foot. This is often the case for post polio patients who show a markedly pronated foot. The abnormal finding is a prolonged distal latency recorded at the abductor hallucis muscle. Stimulation should be above the flexor retinaculum and hence above the site of the suspected lesion. Latencies can be recorded from the lateral plantar nerve also by recording from the abductor digiti minimi. Johnson has reported that some cases show only involvement of the lateral plantar nerve.[51]

Femoral Nerve Entrapment

One of the compression sites of the femoral nerve may be under the inguinal ligament. The method for studying the femoral nerve, reported by Johnson,[49] allows one to determine a latency, from above to below the inguinal ligament, that should be about 1.1 ms. Compression in the area of the inguinal ligament may be precipitated by prolonged squatting, by previous inguinal hernia repairs, and by assuming the dorsal lithotomy position for a long time. If the compression is at the inguinal ligament area, conduction studies of the femoral nerve in the area below this should be normal. Recently, a series of cases with femoral nerve neuropathies secondary to anticoagulation therapy have been described.[54, 68–88] As the femoral nerve descends from the lumbar plexus, it passes through the psoas major and then lies between this muscle and the iliacus muscle. The nerve is entrapped by bleeding beneath the sheath covering these muscles. Femoral compression is also caused by pressure from retractors during certain pelvic operations.[89] Other, less frequent, entrapment syndromes may be found in published reports by Liveson, Spinner, and others.[70, 74, 90]

Peripheral Neuropathies

Nerve conduction studies are an important part of the evaluation of peripheral neuropathies. Two types of processes may be occurring.[91, 92] The first of these is a *dying back* or *axonal degeneration* type of neuropathy characterized by some secondary distal demyelination. The second type of neuropathy is *segmental demyelination* along the entire course of the nerve. In many neuropathies these processes occur simultaneously, with one dominant and the other secondary.[93] These two major changes have the following effects on nerve conduction: In axonal degeneration and the distal dying back phenomenon, the primary change is a decrease in the amplitude of response, while the primary change in segmental demyelination is a slowing of nerve conduction with a secondary decrease in the amplitude of response. Since, in fact, many neuropathies combine both of these features, decreased amplitudes and slowing of conduction may both be seen in many peripheral neuropathies.

One of the most common classifications of neuropathies is based on etiology. For example, diabetes would be included under the heading of endocrine and systemic neuropathies. Patients with chronic diabetes often demonstrate symmetric distal peripheral neuropathy in which the major involvement is sensory. Conduction studies in diabetic individuals demonstrate prolonged sensory and motor conduction times.[94] In acute diabetes, the problem of an acute mononeuropathy is sometimes noted. In some of these cases, severe slowing or even absence of conduction may be found in the only involved nerve.

In uremia evidence of neuropathy tends to increase with the duration and severity of renal failure. These patients often show symmetric peripheral neuropathies, with slowing of conduction velocities, more common in the lower than the upper extremities. Some clinicians use conduction studies as a method to determine whether dialysis is adequate in patients with severe uremic disease.[95] Serial studies on individual patients may prove useful even though, as a group, patients with uremic neuropathy tend to demonstrate a slower conduction compared to normal groups of the same age.

In chronic alcoholism, peripheral symmetric neuropathies have often been found. Many alcoholics have mild or subclinical neuropathies. The major involvement is in the lower extremities. Two major changes are noted in conduction velocity studies of alcoholics. First, is slowing of conduction as a group but, considered as individuals, slowing may tend to be very close to normal values.[93] When slowing is present, it is usually more severe in the distal portion of the nerve.[96, 97] Secondly, response amplitude may be reduced. Some people have characterized alcoholic neuropathy as a dying back phenomenon whereas diabetic neuropathy is more likely to be a demyelinating type.[98] Outcomes of several studies on alcoholism have shown that both the dying back phenomenon and the demyelination may be occurring at the same time, with the axonal degeneration phenomenon being more severe.[96, 99]

In infectious and inflammatory neuropathies, conduction velocity tests have been performed on patients with Guillain-Barré syndrome. In these patients conduction velocities are likely to be slow, particularly in the midsegment of the nerve. Some tend to have normal conduction velocities. Kimura and Butzer[100–101] use F wave determinations to look at the proximal portion of the nerve in patients with Guillain-Barré syndrome. Kimura reported that in 8 of 10 patients, F wave velocity was slow in the proximal portion of the nerve, while slowing in the more distal segments was not as evident.[101]

Nerve conduction velocity studies have been performed on patients with toxic neuropathies due to industrial agents, chemicals, and heavy metals. Among the heavy metals, neuropathies due to lead poisoning has been studied more than the others. Nerve conduction studies tended to concentrate on the radial nerve since in adults lead neuropathies tend to affect the radial nerve more than other nerves. Findings in lead neuropathy are primarily motor and not always symmetric.[102]

Among the drugs known to cause peripheral neuropathy, attention has been focused on nitrofurantoin (furadantin).[103] The toxic effects of this drug contribute to a peripheral neuropathy that is usually symmetric, with both motor and sensory nerves involved. Sometimes motor nerves are more severely involved than sensory ones.[104] Diphenylhydantoin (Dilantin), which has been associated with abnormal muscle reflexes and sensory disturbances, may lead to a mild slowing of conduction velocity in the lower extremities of some areflexive patients.[105] The effects of drugs on peripheral nerve function may be examined more completely by consulting the work of Kraft, Cohen, and LeQuesne.[106–108]

Probably the hereditary neuropathy that has received the most attention for its effect on nerve conduction has been Charcot-Marie-Tooth disease. Dyck and associates[109] studied this disease both clinically and electrodiagnostically, and reported a marked slowing of conduction velocity in all major nerves.[109–111] The lower extremities are usually involved before the upper extremities and both motor and sensory fibers are involved. In this disease nerve conduction velocities may be slower than 15 m/s. More information about the great number of hereditary neuropathies can be obtained from standard references.[104, 106, 112–114]

Radiculopathy

In nerve pathology caused by herniated discs in the cervical and lumbar regions, traditional motor and sensory conduction studies have not proved to be of great value. In these instances electromyography is probably the more important test in demonstrating the presence of nerve root involvement. The expectation is that in most radiculopathies, unless they involve multiple nerve roots, motor conduction and amplitude of evoked responses will be normal. In sensory conduction studies, amplitude of response and velocity are unaffected.

The *F wave* and the *H response* are both secondary waveforms that occur later than the muscle action potential. The F wave, first described by Magladery and McDougal,[115] is a small potential that occurs on supramaximal stimulation as a late arriving wave most easily recorded from the intrinsic muscles of the hand or foot. The latencies obtained tend to vary and responses do not occur on every stimulus. When recording an F wave, the time base of the horizontal sweep must be set so that this late arriving wave can be seen on the oscilloscope. One method of recording the F wave is to use a storage oscilloscope, and stimulate the nerve 7 to 10 times, superimposing the waves. The shortest latency of the F wave that is displayed serves as the latency.

When stimulating over a mixed nerve, the M response is the first response arriving, and the F wave is a response based on the stimulus being carried antidromically in the direction of the anterior horn cell. When it reaches the anterior horn cell, the impulse is reflected, travels back down the motor axon to the muscle, causing a small second response.[100, 101] Kimura and Butzer have reported using the F wave conduction velocity in the Guillain-Barré syndrome to assess the nerve segment between a site of stimulation in the axilla and the spinal cord.[100, 101] This includes the nerve root segment and provides a way to study some aspects of radiculopathy. This technique is not widely used to study radiculopathy at the present time. Kimura and Butzer also studied the F wave in the peroneal and tibial nerves.[116] F waves have been studied in peripheral neuropathies to examine the proximal segment of a nerve.[110] Velocities may be computed for the F wave in much the same way that they are computed for motor nerves; by stimulating at two sites along the course of the nerve and computing the velocity between the two sites.[115] To compute a velocity on the proximal segment, some authors have proposed using a standard reference point, such as the seventh cervical vertebra spinous process, as a measuring point from the stimulation site on the upper arm or axilla.

The *H reflex* is another late arriving wave first noted by Hoffman in 1918 and discussed later by Magladery and McDougal.[116] The H reflex is considered to be a monosynaptic reflex carried by the Ia sensory fibers, which synapse with alpha motor neurons. The H reflex is obtained through a submaximal stimulus; a supramaximal stimulus suppresses it. The H reflex is most easily obtained from the gastrocnemius muscle by stimulating the tibial nerve. Considerable variation in the amplitude of the H response occurs in normal subjects. The use of the H response to examine radiculopathy has been proposed by Braddon and Johnson in a study of the S1 nerve root.[117] Their report derived a formula for calculating a predicted H wave latency. Goodgold also has reported on the use of the H reflex.[118] Other than this use of the H wave, there are no other conditions in which H responses are reliable enough to be included in most clinical studies.

INTERPRETATION AND REPORTING OF NERVE CONDUCTING STUDIES

Nerve conduction testing is not a diagnostic procedure, but merely an additional evaluation tool very useful for examining a particular aspect of a disease state or injury involving primarily lower motor neurons. Nerve conduction studies should be considered along with the history and clinical findings of the patient.

When reporting the results of conduction studies, several important factors must be kept in mind. The first of these is documenting the findings. This documentation should include the latencies, the conduction velocities computed by segment, the amplitude of the response, and the measured distances on the surface between sites of stimulation, including the most distal site of stimulation to the recording electrode. The distance between the recording and reference electrodes should be recorded. If possible and practical, a permanent record of the waveform should be included as part of the documentation. Simple photographic methods are perfectly acceptable for this documentation.

Documentation serves several purposes: (1) it does give an accurate indication in the record of exactly what was found during the examination, so that if the results are questioned at some future time, there is a documented record to support the findings; (2) in repeated examinations a good baseline of information for comparison is available; and (3) documentation provides a means of grouping data for patients with similar problems in preparation for a clinical report.

Other clinicians who examine a report should understand what the testing practioner considers as a normal value. Normal values for particular equipment and a specific laboratory should be summarized on the clinical evaluation form.

When interpreting the findings of a nerve conduction study, it is important to be sure that the information returned to the referring practitioner is adequate. Interpretations or assessments should be clear and concise. The report should not go beyond the available data and should not be poorly defined. If the findings are borderline and additional or repeat testing is important, this should be clearly stated in an assessment. At times it is useful to refer a practitioner to some relevant literature so that comments made in the assessment can be appreciated. Since nerve conduction testing is not diagnostic, it is important to avoid the appearance of giving a diagnosis when reporting a finding.

SUMMARY

This chapter has attempted to provide brief but basic information on motor and sensory conduction velocity tests commonly used in the clinical environment.

In addition, a wide variety of applications for nerve conduction testing is offered. The material presented should guide the reader to other literature.

REFERENCES

1. Smorto MP, Basmajian JV: Clinical Electroneurography, 2nd edn. Williams and Wilkins, Baltimore, 1979
2. Braddom RL, Schuchmann J: Motor Conduction. In: Practical Electromyography, Chap 2, ed. Johnson EW. Williams and Wilkins, 1980
3. Hodes R, Larrabee MG, German W: The human electromyogram in response to nerve stimulation and the conduction velocity of motor axons; studies on normal and on injured peripheral nerves. Arch Neurol Psychiatry 60: 340, 1948
4. Noback C: The Human Nervous System, Basic Elements of Structure and Function. McGraw Hill Book Co, New York, 1967
5. Dawson GD, Scott JW: The recording of nerve action potentials through skin in man. Neurol, Neurosurg, Psychiatry 12: 259, 1949
6. Downie AW, Scott TR: Nerve conduction studies. Neurology, 14: 839, 1964
7. Sunderland S: Nerves and Nerve Injuries. Edinburgh, Livingston, 1968
8. Jebsen RH: Motor conduction velocity in the median and ulnar Nerves. Arch Phys Med Rehabil 48: 185, 1967
9. Johnson EW, Olsen NJ: Clinical value of motor nerve conduction velocity determination. JAMA 172: 2030–2033, 1960
10. Melvin JL, Harris DH, Johnson EW: Sensory and motor conduction velocity in the ulnar and median nerves. Arch Phys Med Rehabil 42: 511–519, 1966
11. Spinner M: The anterior interosseous nerve syndrome with special attention to its variations. J Bone Joint Surg 52A: 84, 1970
12. Fearn CBd'A, Goodfellow JW: Anterior interosseous nerve palsy J Bone Joint Surg 47B: 91, 1965
13. Warren JD: Anterior interosseous nerve palsy as a complication of forearm fractures. J Bone Joint Surg 45B: 511, 1963
14. Craft S, Currier DP, Nelson, RM: Motor conduction of the anterior interosseous nerve. Phys Ther 57: 1143–1147, 1977
15. Nelson RM: Effects of elbow position on motor conduction velocity of the ulnar nerve. Phys Ther 60: 780–783, 1977
16. Gilliatt RW, Thomas PK: Changes in nerve conduction with ulnar lesions at the elbow. J Neurol Neurosurg Psychiatry 23: 312, 1960
17. Feindel W, Stratford J: The role of the cubital canal in tardy ulnar palsy. Can J Surg 1: 287, 1958
18. Bhala RP: Electrodiagnosis of ulnar nerve lesions at the elbow. Arch Phys Med Rehabil 57: 206, 1976
19. Bhala RP, Goodgold J: Motor conduction in the deep palmar branch of the ulnar nerve. Arch Phys Med Rehabil 49: 460, 1968
20. Carpendale MT: The localization of the ulnar nerve compression in the hand and arm: an improved method of electroneuromyography. Arch Phys Med Rehabil 47: 325, 1966
21. Dupont C: Ulnar-tunnel syndrome at the wrist; a report of four cases of ulnar-nerve compression at the wrist. J Bone Joint Surg 47A: 757, 1965
22. Henriksen JD: Conduction velocity of motor nerves in normal subjects and patients with neuromuscular disorders. Masters thesis, University of Minnesota, 1956

23. Currier DP, Nelson RM: Charges in motor conduction velocity induced by exercise and diathermy. Phys Ther 49: 146–149, 1969

24. Gassel MM, Diamantopoulos E: Pattern of conduction times in the distribution of the radial nerve. A clinical and electrophysioloical study. Neurology 14: 222, 1964

25. Jebsen RH: Motor conduction velocity of distal radial nerve. Arch Phys Med Rehabil 47: 12, 1966

26. Jebsen RH: Motor conduction velocity in proximal and distal segments of the radial nerve. Arch Phys Med Rehabil 47: 597, 1966

27. Downie AW, Scott TR: Radial nerve conduction studies. Neurology 14: 839, 1964

28. Downie AW, Scott TR: An improved technique for radial nerve conduction studies. J Neurol Neurosurg Psychiatry 30: 332, 1967

29. Schubert HA, Malin HV: Radial nerve motor conduction. Am J Phys Med 46: 1345–1350, 1967

30. Humphries R, Currier DP: Variables in recording motor conduction of the radial nerve. Phys Ther 56: 809–814, 1976

31. Echternach JL, Levy F: Motor conduction velocities of the radial nerve, an analysis of measurement errors and related problems. Proceedings, PHS Prof. Assoc Meeting, 1980, Houston, Tx.

32. Johnson EW, Melvin JL: Sensory conduction studies of median and ulnar nerves. Arch Phys Med Rehabil 48: 25, 1967

33. Shirali CS, Sandler B: Radial nerve sensory conduction velocity: measurement by antidromic technique. Arch Phys Med Rehabil 52: 457, 1972

34. Feibel A, Foca FJ: Sensory conduction of radial nerve. Arch Phys Med Rehabil 55: 314, 1974

35. Trojaborg W, Sindrup EH: Motor and sensory conduction in different segments of the radial nerve in normal subjects. J Neurol Neurosurg Psychiatry 32: 354, 1969

36. Shahani B, Goodgold J, Spielholz, N: Sensory nerve action potentials in radial nerve. Arch Phys Med Rehabil 48: 602, 1967

37. LaFratta CW, Smith OH: A study of the relationship of motor nerve conduction velocity in the adult to age, sex, and handedness. Arch Phys Med Rehabil 45: 407, 1964

38. Nelson RM, Currier DP: Motor-nerve conduction velocity of the musculocutaneous nerve. Phys Ther 49: 586, 1969

39. Braddom RL: Musculocutaneous nerve injury after heavy exercise. Arch Phys Med Rehabil 59: 290, 1978

40. Trojaborg W: Motor and sensory conduction in the musculocutaneous nerve. J Neurol Neurosurg Psychiatry 39: 890, 1976

41. Kraft GH: Axillary, musculocutaneous and suprascapular nerve latency studies. Arch Phys Med Rehabil 53: 383, 1972

42. Currier SP: Motor conduction velocity of the axillary nerve. Phys Ther 57: 503–509, 1971

43. Gassel MM: A test of nerve conduction to muscles of the shoulder girdle as an aid in the diagnosis of proximal neurogenic and muscular disease. J Neurol Neurosurg Psychiatry 27: 200, 1964b

44. Spindler HA, Felsenthal G: Sensory conduction in the musculocutaneous nerve. Arch Phys Med Rehabil 59: 20, 1978

45. Thomas PK, Sears TA, Gilliatt RW: The range of conduction velocity in normal motor nerve fibres to the small muscles of the hand and foot. J Neurol Neurosurg Psychiatry 22: 175, 1959

46. Mavor H, Atcheson JB: Posterior tibial nerve conduction velocity of sensory and motor fibers. Arch Neurol, 14: 661, 1966

47. Gassel MM: A study of femoral nerve conduction time. Arch Neurol 9: 607, 1963
48. Echternach JL, Hayden JB: Motor nerve conduction velocities of the femoral nerve. Phys Ther 49: 33–36, 1969
49. Johnson EW, Wood PK, Powers JJ: Femoral nerve conduction studies. Arch Phys Med Rehabil 49: 528, 1968
50. Goodgold J, Kopell HP, Spielholz NI: The tarsal-tunnel syndrome: objective diagnostic criteria. N Engl J Med 273: 742, 1965
51. Johnson EW, Ortiz PR: Electrodiagnosis of tarsal tunnel syndrome. Arch Phys Med Rehabil 47: 776, 1966
52. DiStefano V, et al. Tarsal-tunnel syndrome; review of the literature and two case reports. Clin Orthop 88: 76, 1972
53. Eaton LM: Paralysis of the peroneal nerve caused by crossing the legs: report of case. Mayo Clin Proc 12: 206, 1937
54. Echternach JL: Peripheral nerve lesions following total hip replacement: electrophysiological findings in three patients. Phys Ther 57: 1034–1036, 1977
55. Yap CB, Hirota T: Sciatic nerve motor conduction velocity study. J Neurol Neurosurg Pshchiatry 30: 233, 1967
56. Dawson GD: The relative excitability and conduction velocity of sensory and motor nerve fibers in man. J Physiol 131: 436, 1956
57. Behse F, Buchthal F: Normal sensory conduction in the nerves of the leg in man. J Neurol Neurosurg Psychiatry 34: 404, 1971
58. DiBenedetto M: Sensory nerve conduction in lower extremities. Arch Phys Med Rehabil 51: 253, 1970
59. Schuchmann JA: Sural nerve conduction: a standardized technique. Arch Phys Med Rehabil 58: 166, 1977
60. Cape CA: Sensory nerve action potentials of the peroneal, sural and tibial nerves. Am J Phys Med 50: 220, 1971
61. Butler ET, Johnson EW, Kay ZA: Normal conduction velocity in the lateral femoral cutaneous nerve. Arch Phys Med Rehabil 55: 31, 1974
62. Ertekin C: Saphenous nerve conduction in man. J Neurol Neurosurg Psychiatry 32: 530, 1969
63. Stohr M, Schumm F, Ballier R: Normal sensory conduction in the saphenous nerve in man. Electroencephalogr Clin Neurophysiol 44: 172, 1978
64. Brown E, Arno S, Twedt DC: Bells palsy: nerve conduction and recovery time. Phys Ther 50: 799–807, 1970
65. Coffey GH: Pertinent criteria for electrodiagnostic and clinical evaluation of Bell's palsy. Milit Med 135: 904–908, 1970
66. Waylonis GW, Johnson EW: Facial nerve conduction delay. Arch Phys Med Rehabil 45: 539, 1964
67. Echternach JL: Electrophysiological testing in facial nerve dysfunction. Phys Ther 54: 843–849, 1974
68. Alford BR, et al Diagnostic tests of facial nerve function. Otolaryngol Clin North Am 7: 331, 1974
69. Johnson EW, Waylonis GW: Facial nerve conduction delay in patients with diabetes mellitus. Arch Phys Med Rehabil 45: 131, 1964
70. Staal A: The entrapment neuropathies. In: Handbook of Clinical Neurology, Vol 7, eds. Vinken PJ, Bruyn GW: Amsterdam, North-Holland, 1970
71. Melvin J, Burnett C, Johnson E: Median nerve conduction in pregnancy. Arch Phys Med Rehabil 50: 75, 1969

72. Tompkins D: Median neuropathy in the carpal tunnel caused by tumor-like conditions. J Bone Joint Surg (Br) 50B:809, 1968
73. Kopell HP, Goodgold J: Clinical and electrodiagnostic features of carpal tunnel syndrome. Arch Phys Med Rehabil 49:371, 1968
74. Spinner M: Injuries to the Major Branches of Peripheral Nerves of the Forearm. WB Saunders, Philadelphia, 1972
75. Simpson JA: Electrical signs in the diagnosis of carpal tunnel and related syndromes. J Neurol Neurosurg Psychiatry 19:275, 1956
76. Caldwell JW, Crane CR, Krusen EM: Nerve conduction studies; an aid in the diagnosis of the thoracic outlet syndrome. South Med J 64:210, 1971
77. Daube JR: Nerve conduction studies in the thoracic outlet syndrome Neurology (Minn) 25:347, 1975
78. Sadler TR Jr, Hainer WG, Twombley G: Thoracic outlet compression; application of positional arteriographic and nerve conduction studies. Am J Surg 130:704, 1975
79. Gilliatt RW: Thoracic outlet compression syndrome. Br Med J 1: 1274, 1976
80. Trojaborg W: Rate of recovery in motor and sensory fibres of the radial nerve; clinical and electrophysioloical aspects. J Neurol Neurosurg Psychiatry 33:625, 1970
81. Spinner M: The Arcade of Frohse and its relationship to posterior interosseous nerve paralysis. J Bone Joint Surg (Br) 50B:809, 1968
82. Capener N: The vulnerability and the posterior interosseous nerve of the forearm; a case report and an anatomical study. J Bone Joint Surg (Br) 48B:770, 1966
83. DiBenedetto M.: Posterior interosseous branch of the radial nerve; conduction velocities. Arch Phys Med Rehabil 53:266, 1972
84. Hayden JB: Evaluation of a peripheral nerve injury. Phys Thr 48:1238–1243, 1968
85. Johnson E W, Vittands IJ: Nerve injuries in fractures of the lower extremity. Minn Med 52:627, 1969
86. Sinclair RH, Pratt JH: Femoral neuropathy after pelvic operation. Am J Obstet Gynecol. 112:404, 1972
87. Spiegel PC, Meltzer JL: Femoral-nerve neuropathy secondary to anticoagulation: report of a case. J Bone Joint Surg 56A:425, 1974
88. Young MR, Norris JW: Femoral neuropathy during anticoagulation therapy. Neurology (Minn) 26:1173, 1976
89. Biemond A: Femoral neuropathy. In: Handbook of Clinical neurology, vol 8, eds. Vinken PJ, Bruyn GW. Amsterdam, North-Holland, 1970
90. Liveson JH, Spielholtz NI: Peripheral Neurology: Case Studies in Electrodiagnosis. Philadelphia, FA Davis, 1979
91. Sumner AJ, Ashbury AK: Physiological studies of the dying-back phenomenon. Muscle stretch afferents in acrylamide neuropathy. Brain 98:91–101, 1975
92. Ochoa J, Fowler TJ, Gilliatt RW: Anatomical changes in peripheral nerves compressed by a pneumatic tourniquet. J Anat 113:433, 1972
93. Taylor R: Clinical electroneurographic analysis of alcoholic neuropathy unpublished thesis submitted to old Dominion University, 1977
94. Mulder DW, Lambert EH, Bastron JA, et al: The neuropathies associated with diabetes mellitus: a clinical and electromyographic study of 103 diabetic patients. Neurology (Minn) 11:275–284, 1961
95. Jebsen RH, Tenchoff H, Honet JC: Natural history of uremic polyneuropathy and effects of dialysis. N Engl J Med 277:327, 1967
96. Blackstock E, Rusworth G, Guth D: Electrophysiological studies in alcoholism. J Neurol Neurosurg Psychiatry 35: 326–334, 1972

97. Mawdsley C, Mayer RF: Nerve conduction in alcoholic polyneuropathy. Brain 88: 335–356, 1965

98. Coers C, Hildebrand J: Latent neuropathy in diabetes and alcoholism. Neurology 15: 19–38, 1965

99. Casey EB, Lequesne PM: Alcoholic Neuropathy, In: New Developments in Electromyography and Clinical Neurophysiology, ed. Desmedt JE. Basel, Karger, 1973, pp 279–285

100. Kimura J, Butzer JF, Van Allen MW: F-wave conduction velocity between axilla and spinal cord in the Guillain-Barre syndrome. Trans Am Neurol Assoc 99:52, 1974

101. Kimura J, Butzer JF: F-wave conduction velocity in Guillain-Barre syndrome; assessment of nerve segment between axilla and spinal cord Arch Neurol 32:524, 1975

102. Oh SJ: Lead neuropathy: case report Arch Phys Med Rehabil 56:312, 1975

103. Honet JC: Electrodiagnostic study of a patient with peripheral neuropathy after nitrofurantoin therapy. Arch Phys Med Rehabil 48:209, 1968

104. Goodgold J, Eberstein A: Electrodiagnosis of Neuromuscular Diseases, 2nd edn. Williams and Wilkins, Baltimore, 1978

105. Lovelace RE, Horwity SJ: Peripheral neuropathy in long term diphenylhydantoin therapy. Arch Neurol 18:69, 1968

106. Kraft GH, Peripheral Neuropathies Chap 8. In: Practical Electromyography, ed. Johnson EW. Baltimore Williams and Wilkins, 1980

107. Cohen MM: Toxic neuropathy. In: Handbook of Clinical Neurology, vol 7, eds. Vinken PT, Bruyn GW. North-Holland, Amsterdam, 1970

108. LeQuesne PM: Iatrogenic neuropathies. In: Handbook of Clinical Neurology, vol 7, eds. Vinken PT, Bruyn GW. North-Holland, Amsterdam, 1970

109. Dyck PJ, Lambert EH: Lower motor and primary sensory neuron diseases with peroneal muscular atrophy, Part I and Part II. Arch Neurol 18:603–618, Part I; 619–625, Part II, 1968

110. Amick LD, Lemmi H : Electromyographic studies of peroneal nerve atrophy. Arch Neurol 9: 273–284, 1963

111. Myrianthoupoulos NC, Lance MH, Silverberg DH, et al. Nerve Conduction and other studies in families with Charcot-Marie-Tooth disease. Brain 87: 589–608, 1964

112. Bradley WG: Disorders of Peripheral Nerves. Oxford, Blackwell, 1974

113. Brooke MH: A Clinician's View of Neuromuscular Disease. Baltimore, William and Wilkins, 1977

114. Smorto MR, Basmajian JV: Electrodiagnosis, A Handbook for Neurologists. Hagerstown, Maryland, Harper and Row, 1977

115. Magladery JW, McDougal DB: Electrophysiological Studies of Nerve and Reflex Activity in Normal Man. I. Identification of Certain Reflexes in the Electromyogram and the Conduction Velocity of Peripheral Nerve Fibres. Bull Johns Hopkins Hosp 86: 265, 1950

116. Kimura J, Bosch P, Lindsay GM: F-wave conduction velocity in the central segment of the peroneal and tibial nerves. Arch Phys Med Rehabil 56:492, 1975

117. Braddom RI, Johnson EW: Standardization of H reflex and diagnostic use in S_1 radiculopathy. Arch Phys Med Rehabil 55:161, 1974

118. Goodgold J: H reflex. Arch Phys Med Rehabil 57: 407, 1976

5 | Applications of Iontophoresis

Donna C. Boone

INTRODUCTION

Iontophoresis is the introduction of various ions into tissues through the skin by electricity.[1] Commonly called ion transfer, iontophoresis was described by LeDuc over 70 years ago in an investigation of the transport of chemicals across a membrane using an electric current as the driving force.[2] Since the time of that original description, iontophoresis has experienced periods of inclines and declines in its use as a physical therapeutic technique.

During the past decade, the chief proponents of iontophoresis have come from the fields of dentistry, dermatology, and otolaryngology rather than from physical therapy. In a 1971 survey of 302 physical therapy facilities in the United States, physical therapists in 79 facilities reported using the technique but only 6 used iontophoresis on more than 5 percent of their patients.[3] Vasodilators, local anesthetics, astringents, and enzymes affecting tissue permeability were the most commonly used medications in the facilities surveyed. Conditions for which iontophoresis was administered included: neck and low back pain, arthritis, fungus infections, bursitis, plantar warts, skin ulcers, and other skin conditions.

The physical therapists' loss of interest in iontophoresis may be a reflection of the inconvenience of traditional iontophoretic procedures, the increased use of invasive modes of administration that provide greater accuracy in dosage, and a paucity of well-documented clinical studies that would clearly delineate the most appropriate and effective use of this technique. However, "the virtual elimination of systemic toxicity combined with a locally high drug concentration makes the technique attractive."[4]

The purposes of this chapter are: (a) to present the basic mechanisms of iontophoresis; (b) to discuss factors governing the permeability of skin and membranes; (c) to present information about drug conductivity and tissue penetration; (d) to review recent uses of iontophoresis and the conditions for which it is used; and (e) to encourage more physical therapists to take a greater interest in iontophoresis in view of its systemic safety.

BASIC MECHANISMS OF IONTOPHORESIS

A direct current passing through an electrolytic solution causes ions—electrically charged particles dissolved or suspended in solution—to migrate according to their electrical charge. Positive ions are repelled by a positive pole of the current source and attracted by the negative pole. Negative ions are repelled by the negative pole of the current source and attracted by the positive pole.

Passage of the current depends upon this ionic migration, called electrophoresis.[5] Iontophoresis takes advantage of the ionization state of a drug to push charged particles past biologic membranes. The charge on the particle is directly related to the chemical nature of the surface of the particle.[6] That nature stems from chemical reactions or ionization in which positively charged hydrogen ions are distributed between the surface of the particle and the liquid.

The force that acts to move the particle is determined by the strength of the electric field and tissue resistance. A potential difference is established between an active and an inactive electrode. The electrical field, which causes ion migration, is the gradient of the potential difference and may be expressed by applying Ohm's law.[7] That law is expressed as $E = IR$, where E is the voltage measured between the terminals, I is the current flowing through a resistance in amperes, and R is the resistance in ohms.[8]

Current flows from the positive to the negative terminal. Negative ions flow from the negative to the positive terminal; positive ions flow in the same direction as the current. The amount of current flowing through the circuit will depend on the resistance of the body pathway.[6] This resistance is compensated for by a variable voltage control in direct current generators. The applied voltage is adjusted as required to achieve a predetermined current density.

The density of the current, carried by the species of ion or the amount of charge it carries through a unit of area perpendicular to the current per unit time, is equal to the density of the charge times the average velocity of the ions.[7] The velocity is the product of the mass of the particles and their acceleration and is equal to the sum of the forces acting on the particle. Velocity is a function of current density and distance from the electrode. In a constant electric field, a charged particle moves through a linear medium with a constant velocity. However, the absolute (linear) velocity of the ion differs from its velocity in tissues.[5]

Density of the ion is uniform in the entire region invaded by it.[7] The volume distribution of the ion is proportional to the cube root of the product of the current density and the time of its application. The amount of time taken for an ion to reach a location in the tissue is proportional to the distance traveled.

The path of current through body tissues starts at the tip of the electrode, fans out through the conducting material between the two electrodes, and terminates at the edge of the conduction material.[6] The shape of the conducting path near one electrode is not strongly influenced by the geometry at the other end of the path. Therefore, electrochemical activity in the region of the active electrode is not readily influenced by the placement of the inactive electrode.

Differential tissue concentration of radioactive material (^{45}Ca, ^{131}I, ^{32}P, and ^{24}Na), introduced by iontophoresis, showed clearly that the tissue between electrodes had no greater uptake than did remote tissues.[9] The transmitted ion did not follow the path of the electric current between the two electrodes but concentrated superficially at the driving electrode and was then systemically distributed. Distribution of ions, delivered by iontophoresis into the tissues of rats closely resembled the distribution of ions when another mode of introduction, such as subcutaneous injection, was used.

DRUG SELECTION

Because cellular components are surrounded by membranes of relatively high resistance, most of the current applied to tissues is carried by extracellular ions.[7] All cell membranes have three sites of resistance: water-membrane or water-lipoid, interior of the membrane or water, and membrane-water or lipoid-water.[10] As the ionic material is taken up by cellular components, changes may occur in specific extracellular resistance, in the width of extracellular spaces, and in the permeability of the cell membrane.

In order for a compound to physiologically penetrate a membrane, it must be soluble in both fat and water (biphasic). The water (polar) factor is necessary for good ion formation in solution, and the fat (nonpolar) factor is necessary for good tissue penetration and permeability. During tissue permeation, each polar group (for example, OH or COOH) forms one hydrogen bond with water.[10] To enter fat, each of these hydrogen bonds must be broken simultaneously. Energy is required for the bonds to break. Less kinetic energy is required and greater penetration of fat occurs with molecules with the least number of OH groups. All nonpolar groups (for example, CH_3, C_2H_5) must rupture from fat at the same time when the molecule passes into the water phase. Greater penetration of the water site of resistance will result by molecules with the least number of CH_3 groups.

The ideal compound for iontophoresis is a balanced polar-nonpolar compound with few OH or CH_3 groups and with a high oil-water partition coefficient.[6] Virtually all hydrochloride solutions of therapeutic drugs contain positive ions capable of iontophoresis with a positive electrode. Such drugs include local anesthetics, corticosteriods, antibiotics, vasoconstrictors, and some anticancer agents.

The drug carrier fluid must be considered as well. Ions that compete with drug ions for transfer should be kept at very low levels. The fluid should totally wet the treatment area without forming bubbles at the skin/fluid interface, it should be chemically stable but inert, and it should be nonallergenic. Staining agents, oils, particles, or other ingredients that are messy or could alter conductivity should be absent.

Experiments have determined the most desirable carrier fluids for 1 percent, 2 percent, 4 percent, and 10 percent lidocaine hydrochloride.[11] The characteristics evaluated included wetability, viscosity, thixotropicity, inertness, shelf life, stability, and appearance. Carrier gels were developed using silica gel, hydroxymethyl cellulose, polyoxyethylene glycol, and water. After many experiments in which alternative concentrations of lidocaine hydrochloride and various carrier solutions were used, the most desirable selection was a commercially available 4 percent solution of lidocaine hydrochloride (Xylocaine, 4 percent Topical Solution*), which contained distilled water, antibacterial agents, and a very small concentration of sodium hydroxide for pH adjustment.

Commercially available conductive gels have been used for the inactive electrode.

Selection of drugs appropriate for iontophoresis must take into consideration the electrical characteristics of the drugs. Conductivity characteristics of various drugs necessary for proper conditions of use are documented in the study of Gangerosa and associates.[4] The results of that study are summarized in the following paragraphs, however, reades are urged to obtain the complete report for reference. The suitability of drugs, other than those included in this study should be determined by similar conductivity measurements before the drugs are used as iontophoretic medications.

The drugs included in this study were those of practical and theoretical usefulness with iontophoresis as the administration method. They included: (1) local anesthetics: lidocaine hydrochloride, procaine hydrochloride, cocaine hydrochloride, bupivicaine hydrochloride, mepivacaine hydrochloride, and prilocaine hydrochloride; (2) vasoconstrictors: epinephrine bitartrate, levarterenol bitartrate, and phenylephrine hydrochloride; (3) corticosteroids: hydrocortisone sodium succinate, methylprednisolone sodium succinate, and hydrocortisone sodium phosphate; (4) anticancer drugs: methotrexate, cyclophosphamide, bleomycin, and doxorubicin; (5) nucleotides: adenosine 5'-monophosphate (AMP), adenosine 5'-diphosphate (ADP), adenosine 5'-triphosphate (ATP), adenosine 3',5'-cyclic monophosphate (cAMP), uridine 5'-diphosphate (UDP), uridine 5'-triphosphate (UTP), and thymidine 5'-monophosphate (TMP); (6) antiviral agents: idoxuridine, vidarabine, thymine arabinoside, vidarabine monophosphate, and phosphonoacetic acid.

A lectro MHO-meter equipped with a conductivity measuring cell and a pH millivolt meter were used. The procedures for measuring conductivity of all of the chemicals are well described in the article. The conductivity of sodium chloride dissolved in double-distilled water was used as the standard for comparison.

The specific conductivities of the local anesthetics, tested at a concentration of 10 mM, ranged from 800 to 900 μmhos/cm. With the exception of bupivicaine hydrochloride, all of the anesthetics had a specific conductivity greater than that of the sodium chloride solution (5 mM concentration).

---

*Astra Pharmaceuticals, Worcester MA)

Specific conductivities of two of the vasoconstrictors, epinephrine bitartrate and levarterenol bitartrate, were higher than the conductivity of sodium chloride. The solution of the phenylephrine hydrochloride was slightly less that that of sodium chloride. The concentration of all vasoconstrictors, 0.12 mM, according to the authors, is effective for iontophoresis in clinical practice.

Hydrocortisone phosphate had the highest conductivity of the corticosteriods (concentration 2.0 mM) and exceeded that of sodium chloride. Methyl prednisolone sodium succinate and hydrocortisone sodium succinate were slightly lower in conductivity than sodium chloride.

All of the anticancer drugs showed high conductivities. Two of them, methotrexate and cyclophosphamide, had higher conductivities than did sodium chloride.

Four of the nucleotides were more conductive than sodium chloride. These were the tri- and diphosphates with uridine 5′-triphosphate having the highest. The monophosphates were less conductive than was sodium chloride. The nucleotides were studied because of their relationship to antiviral and anticancer drugs.

Of the antiviral agents, vidarabine monophosphate and phosphonoacetic acid, had very high conductivities. Vidarabine, thymine arabinoside, and idoxuridine, which are nucleoside analogs, had minimal conductivities.

Gangarosa and associates, in the same report, noted that hydrochloride salts of local anesthetics conduct best at a pH of approximately 5.[4] This pH keeps almost all of the local anesthetic molecules in the positively charged form. Increasing the pH tends to lower conductivity by converting positively charged molecules to uncharged molecules.

They commented further that although competition between exogenous ions and drug ions is a negative factor for iontophoresis, the technique still seems to be effective even though some nondrug ions are present. For example, the three anti-inflammatory steriods found to be highly conductive are marketed in solutions containing buffers to attain the proper pH and osmolarity levels. However, successful treatment was reported using steroid iontophoresis.

In general, a maximum drug effect is obtained if the solution contains a maximum percentage of the specific drug ions and a minimum percentage of solvent. The experiment of Molitor demonstrates this concept.[12] In a 1 percent solution of mecholyl chloride in saline, only about one-half of the positive ions were specific mecholyl ions while the other one-half were unspecific sodium ions. When the same amount of mecholyl was dissolved in tap water, which contained fewer electrolytes than saline, the same amount of current transported a greater number of mecholyl ions. When a nonionizable solvent, such as distilled water, was used, the only ions introduced by the current were mecholyl ions. No other ions competed for delivery.

As it is difficult to determine the amount of a drug actually introduced into the body, these determinations are not often attempted. The quantity and distribution of radiolabeled dexamethasone sodium phosphate (D-Na-P) was determined in animal tissue by Glass and associates.[13] Using a Rhesus monkey as the most suitable experimental animal, positive test and matching control electrodes were placed over the elbow, shoulder, hip, knee, and ankle on the left and right sides of the body. The current control module and the iontophoretic electrodes were part of the Phoresor* drug delivery system. The control and the test electrodes each contained 1.0 ml tritium-labeled D-Na-P (approximately 4.0 mg) and 2.0 ml of 4 percent lidocaine hydrochloride (80 mg). A current of 5 mA was applied through the test electrodes for 20 min. The control electrodes were in position for 20 min without current application.

At the end of the current application, the amount of drug remaining in the electrodes was compared with that present before treatment. The amount of drug iontophoresed varied from 0.72 to 1.24 mg or from 19.8 to 31.5 percent of the original approximately 4.0 mg. The amount of drug remaining in the control electrode varied from .26 to 5.8 percent.

Local tissue concentrations were determined from cores of tissue removed from beneath the control and test electrodes of the sacrificed animal. Amounts of drug under the test electrode varied from joint to joint but were in greatest concentration in the skin around all joints. Except at the hip, amounts of drug were detected as far beneath the surface as the cartilage. The local tissue concentrations of D-Na-P were higher with iontophoresis than would be obtained by systemic therapy but lower that those obtained by local injection. Less than 1 percent of the total amount of D-Na-P leaving all electrodes was detected in blood samples.

Iontophoresis (3 mA, 30 min) of radioactive iodide, ^{131}I, was used on a group of human subjects to determine the percent of the applied dosage that appeared in the skin and urine. A control who received 0 mA current for 30 min was included. Radioactivity appeared in the urine and skin of those receiving iontophoresis but not in the control group. From 3 to 10 percent of the applied dose was absorbed.

As cited by Molitor,[12] Bourguignon calculated the theoretical amount of iodine transferred from a 1 percent solution of potassium iodide by a given current. He had first determined in vitro the fraction of the total current carried by iodine ions (transference number). The quantity of iodine excreted in the urine of human subjects during a 72-h period following application was measured. The actual quantity differed considerably from that calculated, leading the investigator to conclude that the transference number observed in vitro was not applicable in vivo.

Molitor[12] repeated the experiments of Bourguignon using an electrolytic solution of mecholyl. The transference number of the solution was determined in vitro as well as at the skin surface of humans and various other mammals. Varying concentrations of mecholyl were employed and currents from 10 to 30 mA were administered for 1 to 3 h. The concentration of mecholyl in the electrode was measured at the beginning and at the end of each experiment. The actual loss from the electrode was compared with the calculated loss using the in vitro transference number. The transference number of mecholyl found in the electrode solution was .241, and at the skin surface it was .33. Thus the investigator confirmed Bourguignon's observation that in vitro transference numbers are not applicable to in vivo treatment conditions.

---

*Phoresor, Iontophoretic drug delivery system, Motion Control Inc., Salt Lake City, Utah.

In subsequent experiments, Molitor[12] monitored the effects of various concentrations of mecholyl iontophoresis, in human subjects, on blood pressure, perspiration, and salivation. Changes in these variables depend on the concentration of drug in the range of 0.1 percent to 0.5 percent. Between the 0.5 and 1.0 percent level, increased drug concentrations did not produce concomitant physiologic changes.

Thus, for the majority of drugs used in iontophoresis, the amount introduced locally and systemically remains somewhat obscure. Animal studies, such as the one reported by Glass and associates,[13] appear to offer the best approach to answers to the dosage question. However, differences between species must be kept in mind when the results of such studies are extrapolated to humans.

TISSUE PENETRATION BY IONS

As noted earlier, in order for a compound to penetrate a membrane, such as squamous epithelium, it must be soluble in both fat and water. Because the body is composed largely of water, the human skin is relatively impervious to water, preventing it from entering or leaving through the epithelium. Electrolytes soluble only in water do not diffuse, while those soluble in other fluids may permeate.

Skin epithelium consists of proteins and lipids in a state of electric neutrality.[5] Its pores have a positive charge below a pH of 3, but a negative charge above pH 4. Most solutions used in iontophoresis have a pH of 4 or more. Once inside the stratum corneum the ions move according to the laws of ion transfer—negative ions migrate to the positive pole and vice versa.

The sweat ducts are the principal paths by which ions move through the skin.[15] Structures such as the stratum corneum, hair follicles, and sebaceous glands have high electrical impedance and contribute minimally to the overall transfer of ions.

When the permeability of mammalian skin (human, pig, rabbit) to radioactive forms of some common ions was examined, the permeability of human skin was lower than that of skin from other species.[16] The permeability constant of excised, half-thickness human skin to ^{24}Na Cl ions was 0.09 μcm/min compared with an in vivo permeability of 0.16 μcm/min. These figures compared with 20 to 60 μcm/min in the rabbit and 3 to 20 μcm/min in the pig. The permeability of excised human skin was greatest to aliphatic alcohols with a permeability constant ranging from 4 to 100 μcm/min, with the highest permeability for the least water-soluble alcohols. Other electrolytic solutions whose permeability constant was determined for excised human skin were: methyl salicylate 3 μcm/min; tri-n-propyl phosphate, 0.8 μcm/min; and tri-n-butyl phosphate, 0.2 μcm/min.

An important deterent to the penetration of tissue by some ions is the formation of insoluble precipitates.[5] Ions of heavy metals, such as copper, zinc, and silver, form such precipitates. This precipitate formation was studied to determine the penetration of ferric ion in pig skin following iontophoresis.[17] The positive electrode was used to transmit the ferric ion from an $FeCl_3$ gel. Control sites were exposed to the gel but no current was administered through the electrode. Skin sites were prepared in various ways prior to iontophoresis. The skin samples were prepared and mounted for electron microscopic evaluation. Greater penetration of ferric ions was found in the epidermis and even in the dermis in experimentally-treated samples. No penetration was found below the dermis. The author concluded that the stratum corneum serves as a "barrier" semipermeable membrane to ions. A skin potential is generated by the difference in ionic concentration on either side of the membrane.

In the study discussed previously in which a Rhesus monkey was used as the test subject, concentrations of radiolabeled dexamethasone sodium phosphate administered by iontophoresis exceeded the calculated 0.52 μg Dm-Na-P per gram of tissue following systemic administration.[13] the mean drug level in the elbow at a depth of 6.5 mm cartilage was 7.4 μg/g of tissue; in the shoulder at the depth in muscle tissue of 12.5 mm, 5.22 μg/g of tissue; in the hip at the joint capsule at a depth of 17.0 mm, 1.80 μg/g of tissue; in the knee at a depth of 6.0 mm in cartilage, 3.23 μg/g of tissue; and in the ankle at a depth of 7.5 mm in cartilage, 1.68 μg/g tissue.

The vascular and systemic effects of histamine iontophoresis were studied in healthy normal subjects to determine the absorption of the drug.[18] Unfortunately the complete method was not clearly described. Blood flow in the forearm and hand was measured with a segment type venous occlusion plethysmograph. A hand and a foot were placed in containers filled with histamine solution, and the containers were connected to the positive terminal of a generator. Circulation in the forearm was markedly augmented during and, particularly after treatment. The histamine entered the bloodstream in quantities sufficient to increase blood flow in the forearm when the hand was immersed in the solution. Dilation of the vessels in the skin of the face and neck was observed. Some patients complained of headache. The investigators reported that the vascular response was never as great in untreated areas as in the area directly exposed to histamine.

The same investigators compared the vasodilatory effects of histamine iontophoresis with other methods of dilation and found a greater increase in blood flow in the forearm with histamine than with topical wet heat, mecholyl iontophoresis, short-wave diathermy, or ultrasound.

GENERAL TECHNIQUES FOR ADMINISTRATION

Current generators come in many shapes and sizes. Some devices supply only direct current, and are powered by batteries or by house current. In other more complex generators, direct and alternating currents are available. Many devices utilize a constant voltage, which increases the risk of a burn, particularly as local skin resistance decreases. With the voltage held constant and with resistance decreasing, the current density will progressively increase, resulting in skin injury. The damaged area has a lower resistance, so the burn will intensify. Direct current voltages as low as 3V can cause burns.[19, 20] Variable voltage control is needed to achieve a predetermined current flow to prevent injury to the patient.

A reliable current regulator, a voltmeter, and an ammeter should be part of the apparatus. Polarity of the terminals must be clearly marked. A current reversing switch is desirable. Well-insulated wires must be used to connect the terminals to the electrodes. Periodic examination of the terminals and the current reversing switch is recommended, particularly after repairs have been made to the apparatus. Changes in leads, wires, or the reversing switch may alter the polarity of the terminal so that the label of positive or negative is no longer true.

A simple method for determining polarity of the terminals follows. When the electrode ends of the leads connected to the generator are submerged in glasses of saline solution and the current is advanced, a weak hydrochloric acid condition is produced at the anode (positive) terminal, due to the release of chlorine gas. Blue litmus paper will turn pink at that terminal.

Electrodes come in many shapes, sizes, and materials. Ready-to-use, disposable electrodes are packaged as part of an iontophoresis delivery system.* Other electrodes have been constructed to conform to body orifices, such as the ear, or for other special purposes that will be described later in this chapter. Other commercially available electrodes have flexible metal plates backed by rubber or plastic and covered with an absorbent material. In the past electrodes have also been constructed of cotton, gauze, or other porous and absorbent material backed with contact plates of tin, lead, steel, or aluminum. For some applications, the electrolyte solution is confined in a basin large enough to contain the submerged body part, such a a hand or foot.

The active electrode is usually prepared by immersing or filling it with the electrolytic solution and then attaching it to the area to be treated. Confining the solution to the treatment area has presented problems in the past. The messiness of the procedure may have discouraged therapeutic uses of iontophoresis. However, the availability of treatment electrodes with conveniently located, closed medication receptacles opens new avenues for the increased use of iontophoresis. The polarity of the active electrode is determined by the ion to be introduced.

The inactive (dispersive) electrode is prepared with commercially available conductive gels or other conductive materials. The entire electrode assembly is fixed in position using adhesive, straps, or elastic bandages. Uninterrupted contact between the skin and the electrolyte solution and between the skin and the conductive material under the inactive electrode is essential. Air bubbles, wrinkles, or other artifacts that produce uneven contact will prevent the current from being evenly distributed and may create a potential for burns.

Before the electrodes are applied, that area of the patient's skin that will be covered by the electrodes must be carefully inspected for the presence of anesthesia; cuts, or abraded or scarred areas, or for skin eruptions. In general, skin that is not intact or has areas of anesthesia should be avoided. If it is impossible to avoid cuts or abrasions, these defects should be carefully covered with nonconductive material such as petroleum jelly or an adhesive dressing impervious to moisture. Damaged skin has a lower resistance to the current, so that a burn can easily occur.

The skin should be thoroughly cleansed with soap and water and rinsed with

---

* Phoresor Disposable Electrodes, Motion Control, Inc, Salt Lake City, Utah

alcohol before the electrode is applied. Heat or other modalities used before ion-tophoresis has occasionally been encouraged.[21] However, Zankel studied the effect of various modalities on the absorption of radioactive ^{131}I administered by iontophoresis.[22] Moist heat, short-wave diathermy, microwave diathermy and ultrasound, and cold applications preceded iontophoresis. The application of heat diminished the absorption of the radioactive isotope, as measured by urine and skin examination. Cold application did not reduce absorption. Thus, heating modalities for use prior to iontophoresis cannot be recommended.

Explanations of the treatment should be carefully given to the patient, who must be thoroughly instructed to report any pain or burning sensation immediately. The current should be reduced to a more comfortable level. Persistent reports warrant dicontinuing treatment and the skin under the electrode area must be inspected immediately.

After the active and the dispersive electrode assembly have been attached to the treatment areas, the current should be increased very slowly until the desired level has been attained. At the end of treatment, the current should be turned down slowly. The skin under the electrodes must be cleansed, dried, and carefully inspected.

The danger of producing galvanic burns at the site of application is always present when iontophoresis is administered. These burns occur more frequently under the negative electrode (cathode). Burns under the active electriode, supposedly positive, have occurred in patients during pilocarpine iontophoresis at voltages as low a 3 V.[19] When the electrodes were checked for polarity, the leads were found to have been reversed during recent repairs. Thus, the cathode replaced the anode as the active electrode.

An experiment, using a volunteer, was staged in the same testing laboratory to determine the cause of the burns. When pilocarpine was placed at the negative electrode and the current was advanced to 2 mA, the initial 20 V DC fell to 5 V after 5 min. At the start the pilocarpine solution had a pH of 7—a weak base—but at the end of 5 min it became a strong base with a pH of 10. The area under the electrode became painful within 30 s and was severely painful after 5 min. A third-degree burn resulted. When the pilocarpine was placed at the positive electrode, opening and closing voltages were 20 V DC and 12 V DC; the pH remained constant at a pH of 7.

Evidence exists that conductive gels, liquids, and pastes undergo electrolysis in the presence of direct current, and burns may occur.[20, 23] Most of the commercially-available preparatins are rich in saline, which will undergo electrolysis even with voltages as low as 3 V DC. During the electrolysis, chlorine gas, or oxygen, or both are released at the anode. Sodium hydroxide and hydrogen are released at the cathode. The solution becomes strongly alkaline, with the pH increasing from 5 to 10. The alkali gradually destroys the insulating epidermis and causes decreased skin resistance. The intensity of the current in that area increases, and the electrolytic production of sodium hydroxide is accelerated. Cell damage and the subsequent release of intracellular potassium ions may contribute to the increased alkalinity by the formation of potassium hydroxide. The majority of these negative electrode burns tend to follow the perimeter of the electrode plate, where the electrolytic production of sodium hydroxide is greatest.

CLINICAL APPLICATIONS

A long list of conditions for which iontophoresis has been used can be compiled. However, many of these are more effectively treated by other methods or the use of iontophoresis is not supported by objective evidence. The reader who desires a more historic review of the applications of iontophoresis is referred to the writings of Harris.[5] The present review of clinical applications of iontophoresis includes diagnostic as well as therapeutic applications.

DIAGNOSTIC APPLICATIONS

Detection of Cystic Fibrosis of the Pancreas

This test utilizes pilocarpine stimulation to induce sweating. The collected sweat is then analyzed for chloride content. This universally accepted pilocarpine sweat test for the detection of cystic fibrosis of the pancreas first described by Gibson and Cooke in 1959.[24] Other methods, including those using ion-specific electrodes and conductivity tests, have evolved since that time. However, the greater accuracy of the Gibson-Cooke method encouraged the Cystic Fibrosis Foundation to recommend it as the method of choice.[25]

Rosenstein and associates reported 25 false positives and 2 false negatives in 62 patients who were examined by other methods and then were reexamined using the Gibson-Cooke method.[26] Reasons for this low reliability appeared to be related to poor interpretation of test results, technical poblems inherent in using ion-specific electrodes, and the widespread use of these instruments in laboratories where a small number of tests are conducted.

The technique for the use of pilocarpine iontophoresis was detailed by Gibson and Cooke[26] as follows:

Equipment:
1. Direct current generator that allows application of 0 to 20 V, with a milliampere meter on which 2 mA can be read accurately
2. Two modified electrocardiograph electrodes
3. Low-ash filter paper discs, 2.5 cm in diameter
4. Gauze to cover the negative, inactive electrode
5. Plastic sheeting in squares 3 cm × 3 cm
6. Forceps
7. Waterproof adhesive tape
8. Weighing bottles

9. Analytic balance
10. Materials for chloride analysis
Solutions:
1. 0.2 percent pilocarpine nitrate
2. 0.07 N sodium bicarbonate

Procedure:
A filter paper disc is placed on the metal platform of the positive electrode. Four drops, 0.2 ml, of pilocarpine solution are placed on the filter paper. This positive electrode is applied to the flexor surface of the forearm and securely attached with a rubber strap. A few milliliters of sodium bicarbonate solution are poured onto the gauze that covers the negative electrode. The gauze should be several millimeters thick. The negative electrode is placed on the extensor surface and securely attached with a rubber strap. Complete contact must be assured between the skin and the electrodes.

The current is slowly increased to 2 mA and maintained at that level for 5 min. The current is then decreased slowly and the electrodes are removed. The skin is cleansed with distilled water and dried with sterile gauze.

A disc of filter paper is removed with sterile forceps from the previously weighted bottle and placed over the iontophoresed area. The paper is covered with a plastic square, the edges of which are secured to the skin with adhesive tape. Sweat is collected for 30 min. The plastic square is removed and, using forceps, the moist filter paper is quickly returned to the weighed bottle, and the bottle is reweighed.

A description of a method for chloride analysis is not pertinent for most readers and will vary from laboratory to laboratory as well. Persons who are involved in pilocarpine iontophoresis should familiarize themselves with the method used at their facility. Patients with cystic fibrosis will have a chloride concentration of 80 or more mEq/l compared with control levels below 60 mEq/l.

In over 7200 sweat tests, no systemic reactions and no contraindications to the technique have been reported.[27] The exact dose of pilocarpine delivered to the patient has not been determined but an estimated 0.4 mg of pilocarpine is present in the filter paper. An average oral or hypodermic dose varies from 5 to 10 mg.

An alternate procedure used 7.5 cm × 7.5 cm gauze squares instead of filter paper.[24] Four milliliters of 0.05 or 0.10 percent pilocarpine nitrate solution was iontophoresed with a current of 4 mA for 15 min. Collection periods ranged from 15 to 90 min.

Criteria for an acceptable sweat test have been listed by Rosenstein[26] and include:

1. Test in a laboratory experienced in the Gibson-Cooke method.
2. Collect a least 50 mg of sweat.
3. Confirm positive tests with a second test.
4. Repeat borderline tests.
5. Repeat negative tests depending upon the clinical picture.

Contact Allergy Investigation

Iontophoresis has been investigated as an alternative to the traditional "patch" test used with patients evidencing contact eczema.[28] Ordinarily, the patient must wear a taped bandage containing the suspected allergens for 24 to 48 h. During that period the bandage may loosen and become moist or uncomfortable.

Diagnosis of chromium allergy was explored using iontophoresis of isotope-labeled chromium. In pilot studies using guinea pigs as subjects, the skin uptake of ^{51}Cr was up to 43 times greater with iontophoresis than with epicutaneous administration, even at the lowest chromate concentrations. Isotope-labeled sodium, ^{22}Na, was used as a comparison substance. With iontophoresis, the concentration of sodium ions was eight times greater than with epicutaneous contact. Gradual increases in current densities increased the skin clearance of chromate ions in contrast to sodium where clearance was optimal at 2 mA for 5 min. The investigators concluded that iontophoretic administration can be used to complement "patch" testing for the investigation of contact eczema.

TREATMENT APPLICATIONS

Administration of Local Anesthetics

Iontophoresis to administer local anesthetics has been occasionally reported over the past two decades and included anesthesia for dentistry as well as for ear and eye surgery. Recent studies compared the duration and depth of anesthesia using various modes of administration and combinations of drugs.

Russo and associates[29] compared the duration and depth of anesthesia produced by lidocaine and by physiologic saline when administered by iontophoresis,* subcutaneous infiltration, and topical application. A two-factor randomized block design was employed with 27 humans as subjects. A positive electrode containing the drug or the placebo was attached to the flexor surface of the forearm. The negative electrode was attached to the extensor surface.

The current was slowly advanced from 0 to 2 mA over the first minute, to 4 mA during the second minute, and maintained at that level for the remaining 5 min for a total duration of 7 min. Then the current was slowly reduced to 0 mA. A maximum current rate of 0.65 mA/cm^2 was employed.

Subcutaneous infiltration of lidocaine or placebo occurred 3 min after the start of iontophoresis. Topical lodocaine or placebo was applied 6 min after the start of iontophoresis.

To test the duration of anesthesia, the tip of a hypodermic needle was pressed on each application site every 5 min until sensation returned. Depth of anesthesia was tested by placing a suture a full skin thickness at the iontophoresed or infiltrated lidocaine site.

Iontophoresis of lidocaine produced an average duration of local anesthesia of 14.5 min, which was significantly longer than that following topical application

---

* Phoresor, Model PM 100, Motion Control Inc., Salt Lake City, Utah

(2.1 min) or placebo administered by any means. However, lidocaine infiltration produced an average duration of anesthesia of 22.2 min, which was significantly longer than that of lidocaine iontophoresis. Depth of anesthesia was the same for both infiltration and iontophoresis administration.

These iontophoretic techniques for administering lidocaine may be useful for patients with an aversion to the use of hypodermic needles, for inducing anesthesia to the area of an abscess before it was incised, before a foreign body is removed, or prior to cutdown before vascular cannulation for kidney dialysis.

Epinephrine combined with lidocaine has been recommended to enhance the quality of anesthesia.[5, 11] A recent unpublished study by Gangarosa and McGahee, using the same iontophoretic delivery system as that used by Russo, indicated that the addition of 1:20,000 epinephrine to 4 percent lidocaine produces profound surface anesthesia lasting 160 min.[30] This duration is adequate for minor surgery. No significant reactions were found in this study or that of Russo.

Anesthesia of the human tympanic membrane has been safely and successfully achieved using iontophoresis of lidocaine with 1:2000 epinephrine.[31, 32] Anesthesia is required prior to myringotomy or placement of ventilation tubes in patients with glue ear or serous otitis media. Hyperdermic injection of the external auditory canal is painful and requires premedication. It seldom can be performed in children. Thus, iontophoresis has provided a painless technique with no harmful effects, a faster healing time, and with decreased scarring.[33]

Conjunctival surgery has also been successfully performed using the iontophoretic administration of lidocaine and 1:1000 epinephrine.[34]

Although physical therapists will rarely become involved in presurgical anesthetic uses of iontophoresis, they should be aware of this technique because they may be asked about it.

Harris described the treatment of patients with herpes zoster and trigeminal neuralgia with iontophoresis of the hydrochloride salts of cocaine, nupercaine, and procaine in an 80 percent alcohol solution with 1:20,000 adrenalin.[5] Painful areas were covered with gauze pads soaked in the solution. A current not exceeding 1 mA/cm^2 was administered for 20 to 30 min and repeated three times per day as necessary. Great care was exercised so that burns did not occur. Further references were not found to support the use of this technique for these conditions.

Treatment of Musculoskeletal Problems

Silver ion iontophoresis for the bactericidal treatment of chronic osteomyelitis was recently described.[35] Although the bactericidal properties of silver ions are well known, diffusion of the ions from the metallic surface is negligible. Excess ions must be present in tissues for full bactericidal effects. Silver nitrate may be toxic in large quantities and is locally sclerosing. Therefore, a silver anode was used to assure the transport of sufficient silver ions into tissues.

Patients treated by this technique had long-standing osteomyelitis resistant to all prior treatments. All dead bone was surgically debrided and pockets of infection opened in all patients. Systemic antibiotics were administered as an adjunct to iontophoresis. The effects of the silver ions on a large number of microorganisms were evaluated before the studies were started. All of the microorganisms were sensitive to silver, including those resistant to antibiotics.

Two iontophoretic regimens, each with an individual type of electrode and an individual type of generator, were given. In the first regimen, 99.99 percent pure silver wire (.625 mm in diameter) was implanted into a hole in the bony cortex after debridement. The wound was then closed. Teflon insulation on the wire was maintained except for the terminal 8 cm affixed to the bone. A current of 1 μA/cm was applied constantly for the first 24 h after surgery with a positive terminal setting. The current was then reduced to 100 nA/cm and the electrode was made negative to stimulate bone production. Iontophoresis was continued for 6 weeks.

A current controlled generator* was used with settings at 1 mA/cm for bacteriostasis and 100 nA/cm for bone stimulation. The generator increased the voltage as the circuit resistance increased.

In the second regimen, silver-impregnated, conductive nylon fabric served as the electrode. The sterilized electrodes, prepared daily for each patient, were moistened with saline and packed into the wound. The silver nylon was connected to the positive lead, and gauze was packed over the nylon fabric. Current densities of 1 mA/cm^2 of silver fabric were applied for 3 h. The silver packing was then removed and the wound was irrigated with 50 percent hydrogen peroxide in normal saline. Whirlpool treatment was administered following the irrigation. Local bactericidal agents, such as betadine-povidone-iodine, were not used in the whirlpool because they retarded growth of granulation tissue and interfered with treatment. Treatment was given 3h/day for 4 days.

A voltage-controlled generator* was used, which was set at 0.9 V or less and delivered maximum current as established by total circuit resistance. For both regimens, the inactive surface electrode was made of carbon-filled silicone rubber securely taped over conductive cream. The position of the surface electrode was changed daily.

In 12 of the 14 patients, treatment was considered successful. The silver ions seemed to serve as an effective local antibacterial agent with negligible toxic effects and activity against many bacterial types. Substantial amounts of new bone were evident in the roentgenographic evaluation following treatment.

The disadvantages were: the ions were confined to a limited zone of activity and all infected tissue had to be excised before treatment. The authors concluded that further use of the silver–nylon fabric electrode in the treatment of open osteomyelitis wounds appears warranted.

Silver iontophoresis in the treatment of osteoarthritis of finger and toe joints was reported to be effective by Harris in 1959.[5] However, no subsequent reports have been found.

Most of the reports on iontophoresis administered to relieve joint or soft tis-

---

* Ritter Company, Division of Sybron, Inc., Rochester, NY.

sue complaints are based on individual cases or on poorly controlled studies. Frequently, other types of treatment have been given along with iontophoresis so that improvement could not be attributed to any one factor. Relief of symptoms of a suspected myopathy, including swallowing difficulties, hoarseness, and choking sensations, were attributed to calcium chloride iontophoresis.[36] Magnesium and iodine ions were administered without satisfactory relief. Radiant heat, gentle massage, and cervical traction were also administered after iontophoresis. Acetic acid iontophoresis followed by heat, massage, and therapeutic exercise was reported to decrease calcium deposits, to decrease pain, and to increase motion.[37]

Iontophoresis, using a 0.5 percent hydrocortisone ointment to carry the drug, was reported to reduce paresthesia, pain, and trismus in a patient with postsurgical temperomandibular trismus and paresthesis.[38] The iontophoresis was followed by ultrasound administration. Repeated success was reported with iontophoresis of a 3 percent solution of sodium salicylate in the treatment of rheumatic disease.[39] Little objective evidence has been offered to support any of these reports.

Hydrocortisone iontophoresis, using a water-soluble hydrocortisone ointment, was used to treat 100 patients with arthritis.[40] The study was poorly designed, measurements were not quantified, and no data were presented to support statements of decreased pain and stiffness and increased joint motion.

Encouraging results were reported from two preliminary, uncontrolled, unpublished studies using hydrocortisone sodium succinate and lidocaine hydrochloride.[11] Localized regions of tenderness secondary to bursitis and tendonitis of the shoulder, elbow, wrist, knee, and ankle were reportedly relieved with greater success than were small joints of the fingers.

The need for well-designed, well-controlled clinical studies is apparent to identify joint and soft tissue conditions that will benefit from drug administration by iontophoresis. Until these therapeutic applications are soundly based, skepticism and criticism are inevitable.

Treatment of Skin Conditions

Most of the recently reported uses of iontophoresis in the treatment of skin problems are related to the control of idiopathic hyperhidrosis of the palms of the hands and the soles of the feet, a common, often very distressing problem in young adults and teenagers. Topical and systemic agents have generally been unsatisfactory in treating this condition.[41] Ordinary tap water[41, 42] or various drugs[43-45] have been used as electrolytes for iontophoresis administration. Treatment usually involved placing the patient's hands or feet in shallow pans into which the electrodes and solution were also placed. The depth of the solution was sufficient to cover the palmar or plantar skin but not the nail folds. Sheets of copper, tin, or aluminum served as electrodes.

Placement of the electrodes in the same or different pans was varied by one group of investigators.[41] They found that patients were able to tolerate currents of 20 to 30 mA with electrodes in the same pan. Tolerance was reduced to 2 mA when electrodes were placed in separate pans. Current was applied for 15 to 25 min for 6 days per week for 3 weeks. Using tap water as the electrolyte, the duration of anhidrosis, based on 23 patients, ranged from 3.3 to 8.6 months, with an average of 6 months.

Another author, also using tap water as the electrolytic solution, reported using a current density of 15 to 29 mA for 10 to 15 min, two to three times weekly, until sweating decreased noticeably.[42]

Moderate to severe hyperhidrosis has been treated using hexa- or glycopyrronium bromide solutions, compared with tap water.[43] These bromides are quaternary ammonium compounds with anticholinergic properties. For testing, each was prepared as a 0.1 percent solution in distilled water and the test drug or tap water placed in a shallow tray with tin electrodes lying on the bottom. The positive electrode was used to transmit the drug ions.

The patients' palms or soles of the feet were submerged in the solution, and current densities of 15 to 20 mA were used to treat adults while 7 to 12 mA were used for children for 15-min periods. Hyperhidrosis was controlled by drug treatment for a longer period than tap water treatment. Two patients were anhidrotic for 3 months following one treatment. Mean duration of dryness following one treatment was 33.7 days for palms and 47.2 days for soles of the feet. Durations for tap water were less than for the drugs. Systemic effects of drug iontophoresis included: marked dryness of the mouth for 6 to 24 h; difficulty in visual accommodation (one patient); abdominal discomfort and micturation difficulty (two patients).

Poldine methosulphate, an anticholinergic agent, has also been used to control hyperhidrosis,[44, 45] when topical and systemic anhidrotic, other anticholinergic, or sedative agents had failed. One author reported using 0.05 to 0.075 percent poldine methosulphate in distilled water administered at the positive electrode for 15 min at current densities of 15 to 20 mA for palms and soles.[44] Treatment was given once or twice weekly for 6 to 8 weeks to 22 patients. Hypohidrosis lasted 2 to 3 weeks, a longer period of time than found with topical administration of poldine or tap water iontophoresis.

A second author used an 0.5 percent solution of poldine methosulphate in distilled water as the positive electrolyte administered for 15 min at a current density of 15 mA.[45] Axillary treatment was reported as well, using a thick gauze electrode saturated with poldine solution and covered with aluminum foil. Hypohydrosis was sustained for more than 3 months in some patients. The technique had a high degree of patient acceptance. Both of these investigators reported that side effects occurred 15 to 30 min after treatment and lasted for 1 to 2 h. The side effects included eye irritation and dryness of the mouth.

Frey syndrome, a common sequel to conservative parotid surgery, is characterized by localized facial sweating and flushing during mastication. These symptoms may occur in the distribution of the great auricular nerve or other branches of the cervical plexus. In 11 of these patients glycopyrrolate iontophoresis was tried as a control measure.[46] A single thickness of orthopedic felt, saturated with 0.1 percent solution of glycopyrrolate in distilled water, was placed on the face. A medical grade, stainless steel wire mesh covered the felt and was connected to the positive terminal. Current was delivered at various intensities from 0.5 to 1.0 mA for 11 min. When the 0.75 to 1.0 mA levels were used, sweating was completely eliminated for 3 to 9 days. Partial inhibition was experienced for 5 to 12 days. When 0.2 percent glycopyrrolate solution was used, xerostomia increased.

Nonhealing chronic ulcers of the skin were treated with xanthinol nicotinate.[47] This drug is a capillary dilator, promotes fibrinolysis, and increases collateral circulation. Cathode administration of the drug occurred from a sterile electrode that covered sterile gauze soaked in a solution of xanthinol nicotinate in distilled water. A constant current of 5 mA was administered for 10 min. The entire procedure was carried out under sterile conditions.

Local temperature changes were selected as a criterion of effectiveness and was monitored by thermography before and after iontophoresis. An indifferent solution of sodium chloride was iontophoresed for comparison. Healthy and ulcerated skin received iontophoresis administration.

The nicotinic acid produced a temperature rise of 1.5 ° C in ulcerated skin after 10 min and of 3 ° C after 20 min of treatment. No changes in temperature were found in healthy skin, with either nicotinic acid or sodium chloride nor in ulcerated skin, with sodium chloride. When hyaluronidase iontrophoresis was administered to healthy skin before nicotinic iontophoresis, a temperature rise of 1.5 ° C was found. The increased permeability of the skin was apparently induced by hyaluronidase.

Five years' experience of the use of xanthinol nicotinate iontophoresis included the treatment of ulcers of various etiologies: 48 diabetic ulcers, 22 healed; 24 ulcers crural arteriosum, 10 healed; 36 ulcers crural venosum, 31 healed; 22 neurologic decubitus, 18 healed; 12 mechanical decubitus, 10 healed. The technique has been used to increase local circulation prior to skin grafting, to improve inadequate circulation in the graft, and to stimulate healing.

Histamine diphosphate, a 1:10,000 concentration, has been administered to promote healing of chronic indolent skin ulcers.[48] The freshly prepared histamine diphosphate solution was placed in a plastic container along with the electrode, which was connected to the positive terminal. The lesion was then exposed directly to the solution, and a current density of 3 to 12 mA administered for 5 to 20 min, two to three times per week. A 15-min period in the whirlpool preceded each treatment and debridement of necrotic tissue followed each treatment. This regimen was continued for several months.

The authors indicated that the procedure appeared to be effective for healing chronic, resistant, indolent ulcers in conditions such as progressive systemic sclerosis, sickle cell anemia, and prolonged venous stasis. No evidence could be found that the technique was of value for treating ischemic lesions.

The most common reactive symptoms were headache, dizziness, local itching, and swelling. These effects were controlled by decreasing the intensity of the current.

A pilot study, using rats and clinical subjects, was designed to determine whether bactericidal concentrations of penicillin could be deposited through burn eschar using iontophoresis.[49] Intact eschar overlies an avascular area that serves as a potential major source for bacteremia. Effective concentrations of intravenous penicillin does not penetrate the full thickness of the burn eschar.

Sterile gauze was soaked in aqueous penicillin, 5 to 10 mg/ml, and placed under the sterile negative electrode and directly over the burned eschar. Saline-soaked gauze, placed under the anode, served as the inactive electrode. In humans the current density was maintained at 5 to 10 mA for 5 to 20 min. Higher densities, up to 50 mA, were used with rats.

Treatment and control sites included: untreated burn eschar; burn eschar treated with penicillin and current; burn eschar with current only; burn eschar with penicillin only; untreated normal skin; normal skin with penicillin and current; normal skin with current only; and normal skin with penicillin only. After treatment, specimens were taken from each site for microbiologic assay.

The amount of penicillin deposited through eschar by iontophoresis exceeded all control areas by 200 times. Penicillin levels of 91 units/g of tissue were found in humans. Bactericidal levels were achieved not only for penicillin-sensitive bacteria but also for some bacteria that require very high doses of the antibiotic. No side effects from iontophoresis were reported.

Herpes simplex lesions, involving areas of the lips, buccal mucosa, floor of the mouth, the soft palate, and gingival, oropharyngeal and nasopharyngeal areas, have responded to iontophoresis of a viral DNA inhibitor.[6] Cotton impregnated with a refrigerated 0.1 percent solution of idoxuridine-5-iodo-2-deoxyuridine was placed on a pencil-like metal probe connected to the positive terminal. Current densities of 0.5 to 0.8 mA were applied to mucocutaneous areas and 0.2 mA to oral lesions for 10 min. Complete resolution of the lesions was found within 36 h following one treatment as compared with 2 weeks for resolution of control lesions.

Other Therapeutic Applications

Reduction of edema using hyaluronidase iontophoresis was reported by three authors,[21, 50, 51] all of whom used a similar technique of administration. One ampule of hyaluronidase (150 USP units) was dissolved in 250 ml of 0.1 M acetate buffer solution with a pH of 5.4. Absorbent cotton material was soaked in the solution and then wrapped, several layers thick, around the extremity. Malleable tin strips or aluminum sheets were placed over the cloth and connected to the positive terminal. The entire preparation was wrapped with an elastic bandage. A large dispersive electrode, soaked in saline solution, was placed under the back of the reclining patient. Treatment duration and current intensity varied from report to report.

Schwartz[50] successfully reduced limb volume in five patients suffering from lymphedema. These patients received a total of 103 treatments. In an effort to determine whether hyaluronidase was absorbed by the skin, Schwartz injected 0.1 ml of 0.4 percent Evans blue dye intradermally. Greater dispersion of the dye was found after hyaluronidase iontrophoresis than at a control site treated only with direct current.

Reduction of edema in both acute and chronic conditions, including sprains, nonarticular hematoma, hemarthrosis, lymphedema, and thrombophlebitis, was reported by Magistro.[21] Current intensities of 5 to 25 mA for 20 to 40 min were reported. The average total edema reduction was .25 to .75 inches. No significant untoward reactions to the treatment were found.

A group of 16 hemophilic patients were included in a double blind controlled study using hyaluronidase and placebo iontophoresis to relieve extravascular fluid accumulation following hemorrhage.[51] No statistically significant differences were found in skin temperature, reduction in limb circumference, or increased joint motion between treatment and placebo groups. In addition to these negative findings, better control of bleeding episodes through the use of plasma concentrates have outdated such measures as iontophoresis for hemophilic patients.

The conductivity of hyaluronidase has never been determined. The question of possible destruction of hyaluronidase by the heat of the galvanic current has been raised[52] but never answered. In view of the inherent instability of the drug in solution, these factors should be determined before further recommendations can be made about the use of hyaluronidase iontophoresis.

Zinc iontophoresis was reported to effectively relieve vasomotor nasal disorders, such as allergic rhinitis.[53] The nasal mucous lining was sprayed with 4 percent lignocaine, then, a zinc rod covered with cotton, which had been saturated with a 2 percent zinc solution, was placed in the nasal cavity, and the rod connected to the positive terminal. A current intensity of 4 mA was maintained for 15 min. Three treatments were administered at once weekly intervals. Two hundred and ten patients were followed for at least 14 months after treatment was completed. Of these, 129 reported no symptoms, 52 were improved, and 29 were unimproved.

In the treatment of plastic induration of the penis, Peyronie's disease, a corticosteroid was administered by iontophoresis.[54] Hydrocortone phosphate, 0.3 ml, combined with 7.0 ml of a sodium carbonate buffer with a pH of 8.5, formed the electrolyte solution. A felt pad soaked in the solution was placed on the penile skin, the felt was covered with a sheet of tin, and this electrode was connected to the negative terminal. A current intensity of 4 to 8 mA was administered for 2 to 6 min on a 3-week basis. Twelve patients received 12 to 13 treatments with complete resolution of their pain. Placques became softer in all the patients.

CONCLUSIONS

During the past decade, interest in iontophoresis has been slowly renewed as the effectiveness of the technique has been demonstrated by otolaryngologists, dermatologists, and dentists. Attempts have been made to improve the ease of administration by developing delivery systems that eliminate much of the previous messiness and provide better dosage consistency. Well-designed studies have provided evidence that established the conductivity levels of a wide variety of drugs and determined the amount of transmitted drug found in tissue. However, a paucity of well-designed clinical studies still exists in determining the validity of treatment of some conditions, particularly musculoskeletal problems.

Physical therapists should give attention to the chemical composition of drugs considered for ion transmission. The ideal compound should be a balanced polar–nonpolar compound with few OH or CH_3 groups. The drug carrier should contain few ions to compete with drug ions and should fulfill other identified requirements. The conductivity characteristics must also be considered. Pharmacologists, pharmacists, or clinical chemists should be consulted about the chemical characteristics of a particular drug before it is administered by iontophoresis. Specific ions and their charges should be clearly identified.

Selection of a generator must consider the advantage of a variable voltage control that will produce a predetermined current flow. Periodic determination of terminal polarity is advisable. Careful inspection of a patient's skin before and after administration is essential.

Objective evidence has been presented for the efficacy of certain applications of iontophoresis. The pilocarpine sweat test has been recommended as the method of choice for detecting cystic fibrosis of the pancreas. Iontophoresis as a complement to "patch" testing for the investigation of contact eczema deserves further exploration. The administration of local anesthetics by iontophoresis has provided a depth and duration of anesthesia sufficient for minor surgery.

Iontophoretic transmission of silver ions in the treatment of long-standing osteomyelitis provided a new and exciting potential use for the technique. Tap water and anticholinergic drug iontophoresis have offered relief of sufficient duration for patients with hyperhidrosis to warrant their recommendation as effective modes of control. The reported successful treatment of chronic skin ulcers using xanthinol nicotinate should encourage other persons to explore the use of this drug and this mode of administration. Although newer antibiotic medications are used locally, singly, or in combination with other drugs to treat burned areas of skin, the deposition of penicillin through burn eschar using iontophoresis appears to have merit in view of the amounts of drug transmitted to an avascular area.

Although iontophoresis has been viewed with some skepticism in the past, partly because of unsubstantiated claims, significant strides have been made toward establishing a more scientific basis for its use. Scientifically based protocols related to individual drugs are needed to better establish optimal current intensity, duration, and dosage. The efficacy of treatment in terms of specific pathologic conditions must also be established. Hopefully, physical therapists will address some of these concerns in carefully designed and conducted clinical studies.

REFERENCES

1. Thomas CL, ed.: Taber's Cyclopedic Medical Dictionary, 13th edn. Philadelphia, FA Davis Co, 1977
2. Le Duc S: Electric Ions and Their Use in Medicine. Liverpool, Rebman Ltd, 1903
3. Amrein L, Garrett TR, Martin GM: Use of low-voltage electrotherapy and electromyography in physical therapy. Phys Ther 51: 1283–1287, 1971
4. Gangarosa LP, Park NH, Fong BC, et al: Conductivity of drugs used for iontophoresis. J Pharmac Sci 67:1439–1443, 1978
5. Harris R: Iontophoresis. In: Therapeutic Electricity and Ultraviolet Radiation, ed. Licht S. Baltimore, Waverley Press, 1959

6. Lekas MD: Iontophoresis treatment. Otolaryngol Head Neck Surg 87: 292–298, 1979
7. Trubatch J, Van Harreveld A: Spread of iontophoretically injected ions in a tissue. J Theor Biol 36: 355–366, 1972
8. Reiner S: Instrumentation for Electrotherapy. In: Therapeutic Electricity and Ultraviolet Radiation, ed. Licht S. Baltimore, Waverley Press, 1959
9. O'Malley EP, Oester YT: Influence of some physical chemical factors on iontophoresis using radio-isotopes. Arch Phys Med Rehabil 36: 310, 1955
10. Uhde GI: The problem of permeability and anesthesia of the tympanic membrane. Arch Otolaryngol 66:391–407, 1957
11. Jacobsen SC, Stephen RL, Seare WJ: Development of a new iontophoretic drug delivery system. Submitted to Institute of Electrical and Electronics Engineers, 1980
12. Molitor H: Pharmacologic aspects of drug administration by ion-transfer. The Merck Report, pp 22–29, January 1943
13. Glass JM, Stephen RL, Jacobsen SC: The quantity and distribution of radiolabelled dexamethasone delivered to tissues by iontophoresis. Int J Dermatol 19:519–525, 1980
14. Zankel HT, Gross RH, Kamin H: Iontophoresis studies with a radioactive tracer. Arch Phys Med Rehabil 40:193–197, 1959
15. Johnson C, Shuster S: The patency of sweat ducts in normal looking skin. Br J Dermatol 83: 367, 1970
16. Tregear RT: The permeability of mammalian skin to ions. J Invest Dermatol 46: 16–23, 1966
17. Gadsby PD: Visualization of the barrier layer through iontophoresis of ferric ions. Med Instrum 13:281–283, 1979
18. Abramson DI, Tuck, S, Zayas AM, et al: Vascular responses produced by histamine by ion transfer. J Appl Physiol 18: 305–310, 1963
19. Jarvis CW, Voita DA: Low voltage skin burns. Pediatrics 48: 831–32, 1971
20. Leeming MN, Cole R Jr, Howland WS: Low voltage direct current burns. JAMA 214: 1681–84, 1970
21. Magistro CM: Hyaluronidase by iontophoresis. Phys Ther 44:169–175, 1964
22. Zankel HT: Effect of physical modalities upon radioactive I^{131} iontophoresis. Arch Phys Med Rehabil 44:93–97, 1963
23. Borrie P, Fenton J: Buzzer ulcers. Br Med J 2:151, 1966
24. Gibson LE, Cooke RE: A test for concentration of electrolytes in sweat in cystic fibrosis of the pancreas utilizing pilocarpine by iontophoresis. Pediatrics 23: 545–549, 1959
25. Report of the committee for a study for evaluation of testing for cystic fibrosis. J Pediatr 88:711–748, 1976
26. Rosenstein BJ, Langbaum TS, Gordes E, et al: Cystic fibrosis problems encountered with sweat testing. JAMA 240:1987–88, 1978
27. Shwachman H, Mahmoodian A: Pilocarpine iontophoresis sweat testing results of seven years' experience. Bibl Paediatr 86:158–182, 1967
28. Wahlberg JE: Skin clearance of iontophoretically administered chromium Cr^{51} and sodium Na^{22} ions in the guinea pig. Acta Dermato-Venereol 50: 255–262, 1970
29. Russo J Jr, Lipman AG, Comstock TJ, et al: Lidocaine anesthesia: Comparison of iontophoresis, injection, and swabbing. Am J Hosp Pharm 37: 843–847, 1980
30. Gangarosa LP Sr, McGahee D: Personal Communication
31. Comeau M, Brummett R: Anesthesia of the human tympanic membrane by iontophoresis of a local anesthetic. Laryngoscope 88: 277–285, 1978
32. Epley JM: Modified Technique of iontophoresis anesthesia for myringotomy in children. Arch Otolaryngol 103:358–360, 1977

33. (Editorial) Iontophoresis—a major advancement. Eye, Ear, Nose, Throat 55: 13–14, 1976

34. Sisler HA: Iontophoretic local anesthesia for conjunctival surgery. Ann Ophthalmol 10: 597–598, 1978

35. Becker RO, Spadaro JA: Treatment of orthopaedic infections with electrically generated silver ions. J Bone Joint Surg 60-A: 871–881, 1978

36. Kahn J: Calcium iontophoresis in suspected myopathy. Phys Ther 55: 376–377, 1975

37. Kahn J: Acetic acid iontophoresis for calcium deposits. Phys Ther 57: 858–859, 1977

38. Kahn J: Iontophoresis and ultrasound for postsurgical temporomandibular trismus and paresthesis. Phys Ther 60: 307–308, 1980

39. Jorns VG: Iontophoresis in surgical disease. Arch Physik Ther 14:103–109, 1962

40. Paski CG, Moss S, Carroll JF: Hydrocortisone ionization. Industr Med Surg 27:233–238, 1958

41. Shrivastava SN, Sing G: Tap water iontophoresis in palm and plantar hyperhidrosis. Br J Dermatol 96:189–195, 1977

42. Levit F: Simple device for treatment of hyperhidrosis by iontophoresis. Arch Dermatol 98: 505–507, 1968

43. Abell E, Morgan K: Treatment of idiopathic hyperhidrosis by glycopyrronium bromide and tap water iontophoreis. Br J Dermatol 91: 87–91, 1974

44. Grice K, Sattar H, Baker H: Treatment of idiopathic hyperhidrosis with iontophoresis of tap water and poldine methosulphate. Br J Dermatol 86: 72–77, 1972

45. Hill BHR: Poldine iontophoresis in the treatment of palmar and plantar hyperhidrosis. Aust J Dermatol 17:92–93, 1976

46. Hays LL: The Frey syndrome: a review and double blind evaluation of the topical use of a new anticholinergic agent. Laryngoscope 88: 1796–1824, 1978

47. Van der Kuy A, Aarts NJM: Thermographical follow-up during treatment of chronic ulcerations with iontophoresis with xanthinol nicotinate. Bibl Radiol 6: 203–209, 1975

48. Abramson DI, Tuck S, Chu L, et al: Physiologic and clinical basis for histamine by ion transfer. Arch Phys Med Rehabil 48: 583–591, 1967

49. Rapperport AS, Larson DL, Henges DF, et al: Iontophoresis. A method of antibiotic administration in the burn patient. Plast Reconstr Surg 36: 547–552, 1965

50. Schwartz MS: Use of hyaluronidase by iontophoresis in treatment of lymphedema. Arch Intern Med 95: 662–668, 1955

51. Boone DC: Hyaluronidase iontophoresis. J Am Phys Ther Assoc 49: 139–145, 1969

52. Popkin RJ: The use of hyaluronidase by iontophoresis in the treatment of generalized scleroderma. J Invest Dermatol 16:97–102, 1951

53. Weir CD: Intranasal ionization in the treatment of vasomotor nasal disorders. J Laryngol Otol 81: 1143–1149, 1967

54. Rothfield SH, Murray W: Treatment of Peyronie's disease by iontophoresis of C_{21} esterified glucocorticoids. J Urol 97: 874–875, 1967

6 | Evoked Spinal, Brain Stem, and Cerebral Potentials

L. Don Lehmkuhl

INTRODUCTION

An evoked potential is the detectable electrical changes (waveform) recorded from particular parts of the nervous system in response to the deliberate stimulation of peripheral sense organs or their sensory nerves at any point along the sensory pathway. The waveform recorded originates from various neural generators in the pathway being tested. Although observations of evoked potentials have most frequently been made of the sensory system, potentials produced by antidromic stimulation of motor axons fall into the same category. Evoked potentials differ from the spontaneous electrical activity transmitted within the nervous system in that they have a definite temporal relationship to the onset of the stimulus and a constant pattern of response in relation to the neural structures being activated.

During the past 20 years, studies of evoked potentials have established methods for detecting these electrophysiologic events as significant diagnostic tools in clinical neurophysiology. When used with appropriate stimulation and recording designs, the electronic averaging method allows very small brain or spinal cord potentials to be recorded and analyzed in the intact individual. These noninvasive procedures are being utilized more frequently in attempts to determine the functional status of major nerve circuits in the central nervous system. Therefore, it becomes important for members of health professions, including physical therapy, to become aware of pertinent details about how these measurements are made in human subjects and what information can be obtained from such recordings. Before proceeding further, readers should review the following definitions to enhance their understanding of the nature of evoked potentials and how they are recorded.

DEFINITIONS

Electrical potential: the electromotive force that determines the tendency of an electric charge to move, or an electric current to flow, from one point to another; measured in volts, millivolts (1 mV = .001 V) or microvolts (1 μV = .000001 V).

Resting potential: the difference in electrical potential (usually of the order of 50 to 100 mV) maintained across the membrane of an excitable cell, with the inside of the cell electrically negative to the outside of the cell.

Action potential: the electrochemical event associated with the propagation of a wave of depolarization (nerve impulse or muscle impulse) along the length of an excitable cell; action potentials have qualities of amplitude, duration, shape, and conduction velocity, which are determined by the type and physiologic status of the cell along which the impulse is moving. The action potential of a typical sensory neuron has an amplitude of 90 to 120 mV, duration of .5 to 2 ms, primarily monophasic waveform and conducted at 50 to 100 M/s.

Afferent conduction: transmission of action potentials (nerve impulses) over sensory nerves; toward the central nervous system.

Efferent conduction: transmission of action potentials (nerve impulses) over motor nerves; away from the central nervous system.

Antidromic conduction: transmission of action potentials (nerve impulses) in a direction opposite to the normal; e.g. motor nerves conducting impulses toward the spinal cord following electrical stimulation of a peripheral nerve.

Conduction velocity: the speed with which a volley of nerve impulses travels along a bundle of nerve fibers.

Surface electrodes: electrodes placed on the skin overlying structures to be stimulated, or from which the electrical activity is to be recorded; they are relatively distant from the active neural structures.

Epidural electrodes: electrodes placed inside the spinal canal and resting on the dura mater (the tough outer covering of the spinal cord); the distance to the surface of the spinal cord may be several millimeters.

Subdural electrodes: electrodes that penetrate the dura and lie in the arachnoid space.

Intrathecal electrodes: electrodes that penetrate the arachnoid and lie in the subarachnoid space immediately adjacent to the pia mater covering the spinal cord.

Monopolar recording: a situation existing when one of the pair of recording electrodes (exploring electrode) is located in the vicinity of electrical activity and the second electrode (reference electrode) is at a distant, inactive site.

Bipolar recording: a situation existing when the two electrodes are placed relatively close together to record electrophysiologic events.

Evoked potential: an event-related electrical response induced in a particular portion of the central nervous system (e.g. spinal cord, brain stem, cerebellum, cortex) by stimulation of sensory end-organs or afferent nerve trunks.

Onset latency: the time (in milliseconds) between application of a stimulus and the appearance of an electrical response at the recording site.

Signal-to-noise ratio: the ratio of signal magnitude to noise-level magnitude. The signal-to-noise ratio should be as high as possible when measurements of electrical events of small amplitude are attempted.

Summated evoked potentials: the net electrical response recorded when responses to a number of repetitions of the stimulus are added algebraically to enhance the amplitude of the neural response.

Analog record: a continuous representation of the variable being recorded; the electrocardiogram, as it is commonly recorded on a strip chart, is a typical example of an analog recording of the voltage fluctuations associated with the activation of cardiac muscle.

Digital record: an intermittent (numerical) representation of the variable being recorded.

Analog-to-digital conversion: the process by which a continuous (analog) voltage signal is converted to a sequence of numbers (digits) that represent the analog voltage as it varies with time. Two processes are involved in digitizing analog data: measuring the analog voltage at discrete points in time (sampling) and assigning a digital number to represent the analog voltage (quantizing).

Artifact: any component of a recorded signal extraneous to the variable represented by the signal. Random noise generated within the measuring instrument, electrical interference (including 60 Hz pickup), cross-talk between recording channels, and all unwanted variations in the signal are considered artifacts. Sometimes these variations are indistinguishable from the measured variable; at other times, they may be sufficient to obscure the desired information completely.

COMPONENTS OF INSTRUMENTATION

A block diagram of general features of the instrumentation system for recording evoked responses from the human nervous system is shown in Figure 6-1. The basic components of this system include the electrodes for detecting electrical activity in the nervous system, the preamplifier system that amplifies the signal, conditioning elements that filter the signal to reduce the amount of background interference, additional amplifiers to further increase the amplitude of the biologic signal, digitizing and processing components to average multiple presentations of the response, memory and displaying components, and control components to synchronize the application of stimuli with the recorder to capture the evoked response.

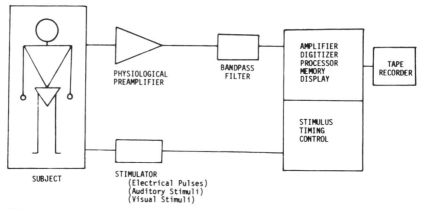

Fig. 6-1. Instrumentation system for recording event-related potentials from various portions of the central nervous system of human subjects. Recording electrodes may be placed over the spinal cord, brain stem or cortical areas, depending on the focus of interest. Sensory end organs may be stimulated with electrical pulses or auditory or visual stimuli.

BIOELECTRIC POTENTIALS

When a cell is excited and generates an action potential, ionic currents begin to flow. In the case of a nerve cell with a long axon, the action potential is generated over a very small segment of its length. As the action potential travels along the nerve fiber, it cannot reexcite the portion of the fiber immediately behind the advancing wave of depolarization because of the refractory period that follows the action potential. However, excitation of a nerve fiber somewhere along its length can produce an action potential propagated in both directions from the original point of excitation. The rate at which an action potential moves along a nerve fiber or is propagated from cell to cell is called the *propagation rate*. In nerve fibers, the propagation rate is also called the *nerve conduction velocity*. This velocity varies widely, depending on the type and diameter of the nerve fiber. The usual velocity range in myelinated nerves is from 10 to 120 M/s.

MEASUREMENT OF POTENTIALS

To measure bioelectric potentials, a transducer capable of converting ionic potentials, produced by ionic current flow, into electronic potentials is required.[1] Such a transducer consists of a metal plate in contact with an electrolyte at an interface that permits an exchange of ions between the metal and electrolytes of the body.

The silver-silver chloride electrode has properties that make it suitable for detecting small bioelectric potentials for many hours without producing a build-up of reactants at the metal-electrolyte junction (polarization), which, in turn, reduce the effectiveness of the electrode. Measurement of bioelectric potentials requires two electrodes; the voltage measured is really the difference between the instantaneous potentials at each of the electrodes.

The exact method by which electrical potentials that are being conducted over nerve tracts or muscle fibers deep within the body reach the surface of the body is not known. A number of theories have been advanced that seem to explain most of the observed phenomena fairly well,[2] but none exactly fits all situations. A close approximation can be obtained if one assumes that the surface pattern is a function of the summation of the first derivative (rate of change) of all individual action potentials, instead of the potentials themselves. Regardless of the method by which these patterns of potentials reach the surface of the body, they can be measured as specific bioelectric signal patterns that have been studied extensively and can be defined quite well. The amplitude of the measured bioelectric signal is the instantaneous sum of all action potentials generated at any given time. Because these action potentials occur in both positive and negative polarities at a given electrode, they sometimes add and sometimes cancel. Thus, the bioelectric potential waveform often appears like a random-noise waveform.

INFLUENCE OF ELECTRODE GEOMETRY ON RECORDED WAVEFORM

The shape and polarity of bioelectric potentials representing electrical activity in particular parts of the nervous system are very much affected by the location of the recording electrodes in relation to the source of generation and the direction of propagation of the nerve impulses.[3] To understand and interpret the record obtained when recording an advancing wave of action potentials, consider the following example: Figure 6-2 depicts the sequence of events following stimulation of a nerve trunk in a conducting medium. A monopolar arrangement for recording is used, with the exploring electrode on the surface of the nerve and the reference electrode in contact with inactive tissue having the properties of an electrolytic conductor. As the impulse propagates to the right, the recorded potential is shown on the screen of the oscilloscope. Before stimulation, there is no external current flow and, therefore, no potential difference between the electrodes; the baseline is at zero. As depolarization at the excited region proceeds, the outward flow of current through adjacent regions of the membrane makes the exploring electrode more positive with respect to the reference electrode; that is, the exploring electrode is situated over a region that acts as a source of current and thus will be at a higher electrical potential relative to the distant electrode. Consequently, the first result of the impulse approaching the electrode is a positive, or downward, deflection.*

---

* In the physical sciences, the accepted convention is to display positive potentials "upward" and the negative potentials "downward." However, in electrophysiology a reversed convention is in common use: positive potentials, down; negative potentials, up. The direction chosen to represent a polarity is completely arbitrary.

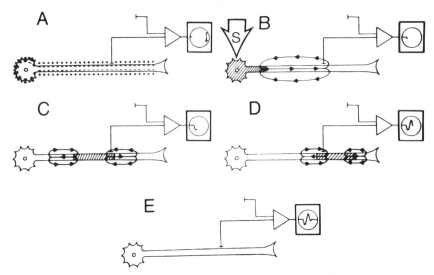

Fig. 6-2. Relationship between the waveform recorded on an oscilloscope and the movement of the action potential over a nerve fiber when using a monopolar arrangement of electrodes. (S = stimulus.) A. Excitable fiber and electrodes immersed in a volume conductor. Monopolar recording arrangement with reference electrode at a distant location. There is no external current flow and, therefore, no potential difference between the two electrodes. The oscilloscope records a zero baseline. B. Depolarization at the excited region produces outward flow of current through adjacent regions of the membrane. The exploring electrode becomes more positive with respect to the reference electrode. The first result of the impulse approaching the electrode is a positive (downward) deflection of the oscilloscope beam. C. Region under exploring electrode becomes increasingly depolarized. Inward current flow causes exploring electrode to become negative with respect to the reference electrode and an upward deflection of the oscilloscope beam is observed. D. The impulse has passed under the exploring electrode and become subject to a field of outward current flow, causing the oscilloscope beam to deflect downward. E. As the impulse moves further along the fiber, the exploring electrode ceases to be influenced by the current flow and the oscilloscope beam returns to the original baseline. The net potential changes detected by the exploring electrode are triphasic in waveform and last a few milliseconds.

A short time later, the region underneath the exploring electrode will be invaded by the action potential and reverse its polarity. The current will now flow from the adjacent regions into this area. The exploring electrode will be negative with respect to the reference electrode, and an upward deflection is observed. This positive to negative deflection is steep in slope and corresponds to the sharp rise of the intracellular action potential.[2] As the area under the exploring electrode repolarizes, the electrode is over a region that acts as a source of current, and its potential is positive relative to the reference electrode. The recorded potential thus progresses downward (negative to positive) from the peak of the negative deflection. As the impulse moves further along the fiber, the exploring electrode ceases to be influenced by the current flow, and the observed potential slowly returns to original baseline. The complete potential change produced by an impulse propagated along the fiber is thus triphasic, with a steep linear positive-negative deflection.

Another arrangement for recording bioelectric potentials is the use of two closely spaced electrodes placed in the vicinity of the generation or propagation of the nerve impulses to be monitored. Figure 6-3 illustrates the type of waveform recorded with bipolar recording. Initially, the electrodes are isopotential with one another, and the oscilloscope trace will register a zero baseline. As the action potential approaches the recording electrodes from a distance, both are "seeing" approximately the same current flow; therefore, there is little or no initial positive deflection (Fig. 6-3B). As the action potential passes under the first electrode, a maximum difference in voltage occurs between the electrodes. When the action potential is midway between the electrodes, the relative difference in potential becomes zero (Fig. 6-3C); when it passes under the second electrode, the potential difference becomes maximal in the opposite direction (Fig. 6-3D); and when the impulse passes beyond both electrodes, the oscilloscope trace returns to the baseline (Fig. 6-3E). Thus, the complete sequence of potential change consists of two more-or-less symmetric phases of opposite polarity (a biphasic waveform). When the electrodes are close enough so that there is no time interval during which the propagating wave is entirely contained between the recording electrodes, the isopotential interval between peaks is reduced toward zero and the falling phase of the waveform passes directly through the baseline to the positive peak.

In these examples, the recording electrode was close to the source of the electrical activity or active fiber. For a given arrangement of recording electrodes, the shape of the extracellular action potential is also determined by: (1) the distance between the active fiber and the electrode, (2) the properties of the fiber, and, (3)

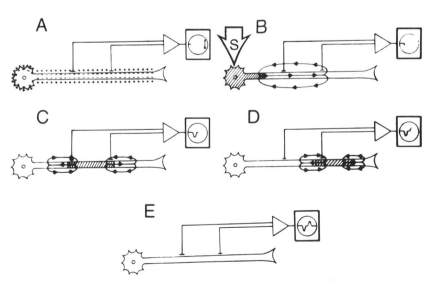

Fig. 6-3. Relationship between the waveform recorded on the oscilloscope and the movement of the action potential over a nerve fiber when a bipolar arrangement of recording electrodes is used. (S = stimulus.)

the structure and conductivity of the volume conductor surrounding the active fiber.

Extracellular potentials recorded at different points along the nerve and at various distances from it are illustrated in Figure 6-4. In this example, the nerve is arranged such that point *a* represents a point on the nerve where the impulse is initiated. If recording electrodes are placed at different points on the nerve at fixed distances from point *a*, we observe the potentials illustrated in Figure 6-4. The reference electrode is located at a distant, inactive site. At point *a*, the impulse travels only away from the electrode so that the first change seen by the electrode is depolarization (negative deflection) followed by repolarization (positive). Hence, a diphasic response is recorded. At points further along the nerve (*b* and *c*), triphasic potentials are observed as expected. However, at *d* a positive-negative diphasic response is seen. Point *d* is the end of the fiber and the third (positive) deflection is missing because there is no current flow from the region beyond the electrode.

If we now place electrodes at different distances from the fiber, we obtain a new set of curves. For example, by placing electrodes at 3 and 10 mm from the fiber, potentials (*e* through *l*) lower in amplitude and slower in positive-negative rise time are obtained. With further movement away from the fiber, the amplitude decreases appreciably and the slope becomes considerably slower. Rosenfalck[5]

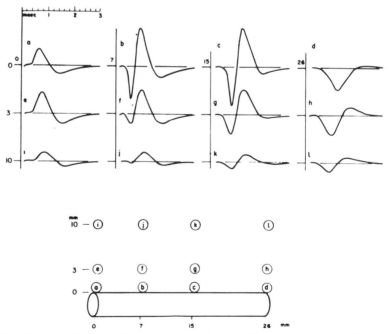

Fig. 6-4. Extracellular potentials recorded with an exploring electrode at different points along the nerve (*a, b, c, d*) and at various distances from it (0, 3, and 10 mm). Impulse is initiated at point *a* and propagates to the right. The reference electrode is remote, providing a monopolar recording arrangement. (Reproduced by permission from Goodgold J, Eberstein A: Electrodiagnosis of Neuromuscular Diseases. Baltimore, Williams and Wilkins, 1972, p 39.)

calculated that the peak-to-peak amplitude of an intracellular action potential decreases 90 percent within about .5 mm from the fiber and continues to decrease exponentially with distance. Thus, for an intracellular potential of about 100 mV, the extracellular potential several centimeters away on the surface of the body is about .001 to .01 mV (or 1 to 10 μV) peak-to-peak.

ELECTRODE ARTIFACTS

Most surface recording electrodes suffer from a common problem. They are sensitive to movement, some to a greater degree than others. Even the slightest movement changes the thickness of the thin film of electrolyte between metal and skin, and thus causes changes in the electrode potential and the impedance between electrode and skin. In many cases, the potential changes are so large that they completely obscure the bioelectric potentials the electrodes attempt to measure. A relatively new type of electrode, the "floating electrode," has been introduced in various forms by several manufacturers. The principle of this electrode is to practically eliminate movement artifact by avoiding any direct contact between metal and skin. The only conductive path between metal and skin is the electrode paste or jelly, which forms an electrolyte bridge. Even with the electrode surface held at a right angle to the skin surface, performance is not impaired as long the electrolyte bridge maintains contact with both the skin and metal. Figure 6-5 shows a cross-section of a floating electrode.

Another source of difficulty in recording bioelectric potentials of small amplitude is the presence of a junction potential at the interface of metallic ions in solution and their associated metals. If the two electrodes are of the same type, the net potential difference is usually small and depends essentially on the actual difference in ionic potential between the two points of the body from which measurements are being taken. If the two electrodes are different, however, they may produce a significant DC voltage that can cause current to flow through both electrodes, as well as through the input circuit of the amplifier to which they are connected. The DC voltage due to the difference in electrode potentials is called

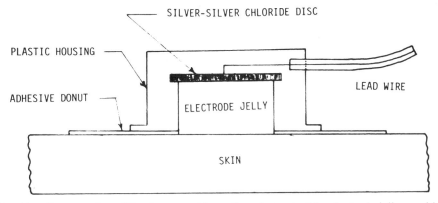

Fig. 6-5. Cross-section of floating type skin surface electrode. The electrode jelly provides good electrical contact between the silver disc and the subject's skin even though relative motion may occur between them.

the *electrode offset voltage*. The resulting current is often mistaken for a true physiologic event. Even two electrodes of the same material may produce a small electrode offset voltage. In addition to the electrode voltage, experiments have shown that the chemical activity that takes place within an electrode can cause voltage fluctuations to appear without any physiological input. Such variations may appear as noise on a bioelectric signal. This noise can be reduced by a proper choice of materials or, in most cases by special treatment, such as coating the electrodes by some electrolytic method to improve stability. Electrochemically, the silver-silver chloride electrode is very stable. This type of electrode is prepared by electrolytically coating a piece of pure silver with silver chloride.

The electrical impedance of an electrode describes the resistance to flow of current between the wire attached to the electrode and the fluids making up the volume conductor of the body. Larger electrodes tend to have lower impedances. Surface electrodes generally have impedances of 1 to 10,000 ohms; whereas, small needle electrodes and microelectrodes have much higher impedances.

CHARACTERISTICS OF RECORDING EQUIPMENT

For recording bioelectric potentials, the electrodes are connected to a preamplifier, a differential amplifier with high common-mode rejection. The preamplifier is AC-coupled to avoid problems with small DC voltages that may originate from polarization of the electrodes. The preamplifier boosts the signal by a factor of 1 to 5, and the output of this preamplifier is fed to another amplifier, which conditions the signal further. Most modern amplifiers include adjustable upper and lower frequency limits to allow the operator to select a bandwidth suitable for the conditions of measurement. In addition, some instruments have a fixed 60-Hz rejection filter to reduce power line interference.

It is possible to obtain amplifiers with gains in the range of 20 to 100,000 and bandwidths in the range of 1 Hz to 10 kHz, while maintaining a noise level of less than 3 μV peak-to-peak; even less, if more restricted bandwidths are used. Precautions must be taken to ensure that any residual electronic noise is not synchronous with the stimulus.

Input Impedance

The input impedance of an amplifier describes the resistance of the amplifier input to the flow of current through the amplifier. Having a high input impedance ensures that very little current will be drawn from the source of the potential to be amplified, and that there is minimal drop in voltage at the electrode. The input impedance should be many times greater than the impedance of the electrode-skin interface.

Differential Input

A differential amplifier is characterized by its rejection of voltages, which are identical (in both amplitude and time) at its two input terminals, and the amplification of voltage differences between the two input terminals. Thus, signals arising from power lines or from sources outside the electrode field, which would normally interfere with the recording of bioelectric potentials, will not be passed on by the amplifier.

Frequency Response

Electronic filtering of signals allows signals (changes in voltage) that fall within a certain spectrum of rates of rise of the signal to pass through the amplifier. Figure 6-6 illustrates the frequency response characteristics for an amplifier.

The output voltage remains constant or "flat" for a portion of the frequency spectrum and decays at both ends of the curve. The points on the curve designated f_L and f_H represent frequencies at which the ratio of voltage output to voltage input is .707 of the midband value. Stated another way, the output of the amplifier is said to be down 3 decibels at these designated low and high cut-off frequencies. Biologic signals such as the electrocardiogram, electroencephalogram, and evoked responses are commonly recorded using a bandpass filter between 1 Hz and 100 Hz. However, recordings made over the spinal cord, particularly those with response characteristics of nerve roots, have much higher frequency content (related to how fast the signal rises or falls) and require as much as 10,000 Hz bandwidths. Using a too narrow bandwidth can result in marked attenuation of the signal and may even result in a phase shift in the response peaks.

Figure 6-7 illustrates the effect of altering the recording system. Evoked potentials were averaged simultaneously from the same signal using three different filters (0-2500 Hz in A; 0-1500 Hz in B; 0-250 Hz in C). Note the loss in resolution of some of the components and the apparent prolongation of latency due to a phase shift of the fastest components.

In selecting the best frequency response for the amplifier, two factors are equally important: avoiding distortion of the signal of interest and keeping noise voltages as low as possible. Choosing a wide frequency bandpass to ensure distortion-free recording may also allow considerable noise to pass through the amplifier. Thus, the filters are selected on the basis of expected rate of rise of the wave of interest and the suppression of other voltage fluctuations.

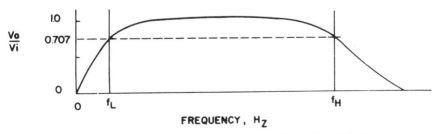

Fig. 6-6. A frequency response characteristic for an amplifier. The high frequency cut-off is labeled f_H and the low frequence cut-off is labeled f_L. Vo/Vi is the ratio of voltage output to input. (Reproduced by permission from Goodgold J, Eberstein A: Electrodiagnosis of Neuromuscular Diseases. Baltimore, Williams and Wilkins, 1972, p 49.)

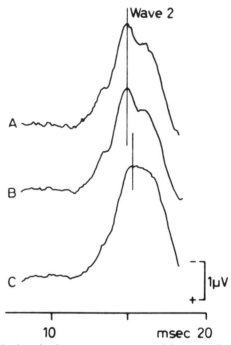

Fig. 6-7. Effect of reducing the frequency response of the recording system. The same responses were recorded simultaneously with different fibers: A = 0-2500 Hz; B = 0-1500 Hz; C = 0-250 Hz. (Reproduced by permission from Small GD, Beauchamp M, Matthews WB: Subcortical somatosensory evoked potentials in normal man and in patients with central nervous system lesions. In: Progress in Clinical Neurophysiology, vol 7 ed. Desmet JE. Basel, S. Karger, AG, 1980, pp 190–209.)

SIGNAL AVERAGING

Signal averaging is a process used to recover biologic signals of small amplitude that are buried in noise. Not all noisy signals can be averaged to obtain a record of the response; there are certain conditions that need to be met for signal averaging to be accomplished. The primary conditions are that the biologic signal be repeatable and associated with a trigger signal that can be used to lock the response on the timebase of a recording device. The timing of the signal is critical for the averaging process to work. The biologic potentials evoked by electrical stimulation of an excitable tissue are particularly amenable to the process of signal averaging because the stimulus artifact can be used to initiate the sweep of an oscilloscope, and the response evoked by the stimulus will appear at the same location along the timebase.

The instrument that performs the signal averaging is a digital signal averager, similar to a digital computer. A digital system is used because it has the ability to convert an analog signal to numerical values at precise times along a timebase. In addition, digital memory is a very convenient way of storing large amounts of information for later processing. The averager is responsible for improving the sig-

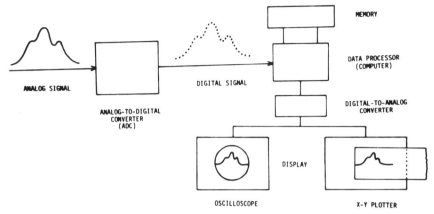

Fig. 6-8.   Components utilized in the conversion of an analog signal to a digital signal for processing and display.

nal-to-noise ratio by adding successive responses together. A diagram of the components of a signal averager is shown in Figure 6-8. The averager consists of an analog-to-digital converter, which converts the incoming signal into evenly spaced discrete samples. These sampled waveforms are then appropriately summed into the digital memory. Also connected to the processor is a digital-to-analog converter, which converts the discrete averaged points into analog voltages for the display oscilloscope and the X-Y plotter.

The key concept that must be understood about an averager is the conversion of a continuous analog signal into a discrete digital signal. Three timing parameters are involved in this process. They are: intersample interval, sweep time, and memory size (number of points).

As a conceptual introduction to discrete sampling, Figure 6-9 illustrates the relationship between an analog waveform and its digital counterpart. The main thing to notice is that given enough points, a waveform can be well represented in digital form. Conversely, when not provided with enough points, the waveform is not well represented.

Horizontal Resolution

To accurately represent an analog waveform the intersample interval must be substantially smaller than the shortest event in the wave. Assume that in Figure 6-9 the major peak is 1 ms long and that 20 points will accurately represent it. The required intersample interval would have to be equal to or less than .05 ms. In short, the required intersample interval is determined by the shortest event in the recording being made.

After the intersample interval has been determined, the sweep time equals the intersample interval multiplied by memory size. Let us take a specific example to illustrate this point. Say that a particular averager has 256 points of memory available and the electrophysiologic events we wish to record can be captured

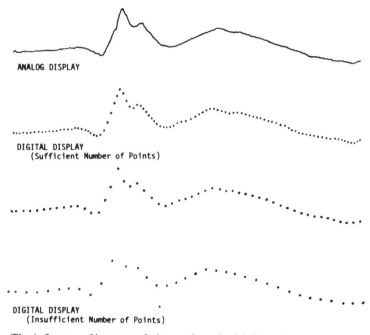

ANALOG DISPLAY

DIGITAL DISPLAY
(Sufficient Number of Points)

DIGITAL DISPLAY
(Insufficient Number of Points)

Fig. 6-9. The influence of intersample interval on the fidelity with which a digital display represents the analog waveform.

within a timebase of 40 ms. However, we wish to record from four different electrode sites, thereby requiring four channels of recorded information. Therefore, 256 memory points must be divided among the four channels, or 64 points per channel, to display events occurring over a time period of 40 ms. An average of 1.6 memory points will be available each 1 ms of timebase. Another way of saying this is that the memory points would be .625 ms apart (1/1.6).

Vertical Resolution

An analog-to-digital conversion involves converting a continuous voltage level to a discrete number. Thus, the size of the A to D converter (number of bites) defines how accurately this voltage may be resolved for the averager. For example, a digitizer the size of two bites has a resolution of one part in four (2 to the 2nd power), and a digitizer with 8 bites has a resolution of 1 part in 256 (2 to the 8th power). Consider a 2-bite digitizer with a biologic signal voltage range of ± 10 μV. The input signal can be resolved to within 5 μV (20/4) of its correct value. A signal that falls between two discrete steps must be assigned to one of them. In this example, this means that input voltage differences of less than 5 μV cannot be resolved. On the other hand, with an 8-bite digitizer the signal can be resolved to within .078 μV (20/256). Summing many sweeps, as is done in signal averaging, will enhance the resolution proportional to the number of sweeps being averaged.

For instance, an average of 100 sweeps will enhance the resolution by a factor of 100.

To summarize, the response obtained from each stimulus is added to those previously stored in the memory. As many repetitions as desired may be taken and the average is then computed. During any given time interval, the background noise in the recording will occur as random events. Therefore, over a long sampling period, there will be an equal quantity of positive deflections representing noise as there are negative deflections at each point along the timebase. Algebraically, summing these voltage fluctuations results in a net voltage that approximates zero. The exception is the appearance of the evoked response at a particular place along the timebase. Each of these responses shows up as voltage changes in the same direction on each repetition. As these responses are added al-

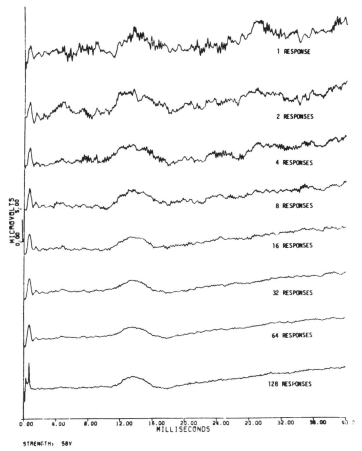

STRENGTH: 56V

Fig. 6-10. Improvement in signal-to-noise ratio of an evoked potential by averaging repetitive responses. The exploring electrode was positioned over T10 and the reference electrode over T6. Single 0.5-ms pulses of 56 V were applied to stimulate the left tibial nerve at the knee, following every second EKG signal (approximately once every 2 s). The number of responses averaged is indicated on the right. The signal-to-noise ratio is significantly improved by averaging 16 or more responses.

gebraically, they sum and become larger. At the end of 64 or 128 or as some similar number of n^2 repetitions, the effect is to produce a larger and larger evoked response and a smaller and smaller amount of background noise in the record. Dividing the net result by the number of responses collected yields the average waveform of the original evoked response.

Figure 6-10 shows the effect of signal averaging when attempts are made to record a 2 μV evoked response. As long as the noise is a random signal, averaging will increase the signal-to-noise ratio. However, if there are noise components that are not random but are time-locked to the averager, these noise signals will be summed and their signal-to-noise ratio will be improved along with signals of interest. The variability of the raw unaveraged signal is inversely proportional to the square root of the number of sweeps recorded. From a practical standpoint, the evaluation of how much averaging is adequate is often accomplished by demonstrating waveform replication.

This evaluation requires two or more independent averages of the same phenomenon which are superimposed on the display oscilloscope so that the extent to which individual peaks and valleys displayed in the waveform are superimposable can be determined (Fig. 6-11).

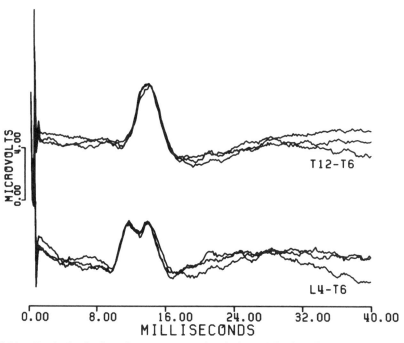

Fig. 6-11. Evoked spinal cord responses to stimulation of the left tibial nerve at the knee recorded from surface electrodes over the spinous processes of T12 and L4. The reference electrode was at T6. Three individual recordings of 128 averaged responses to 45 V, 0.5 ms pulses, applied after ever second EKG signal, are superimposed.

LIMITATION OF THE METHOD

The method of signal averaging is rather vulnerable to a variety of artifacts and interferences that can distort the results, sometimes severely.

Inadequate Stimulation Intensity

Inadequate stimulation intensities can wrongly hint at a delayed onset of an evoked potential. Matthews, Beauchamp, and Small[7] have shown that increasing stimulus strengths produced an initial steep rise in the amplitude of the recorded response and a moderate reduction in latency, both measurements leveling off at a stimulus intensity approximately threshold for a motor response (Fig. 6-12). A stimulus of approximately four times sensory threshold (which, through personal experience, may be quite uncomfortable) is often used for routine recording; this produces a moderate muscle twitch.

Mixture of Orthodromic and Antidromic Impulses

A major disadvantage of passing electric pulses through a peripheral nerve to evoke a response is that the stimulation of a mixed nerve elicits nerve impulses conducted antidromically in motor fibers, as well as nerve impulses conducted orthodromically in sensory nerves. Under some circumstances, the stimulation can be restricted to limited cutaneous areas, which improves the homogeneity of the population of afferent nerve fibers stimulated. However, with this procedure the amplitude of the evoked response is markedly reduced.

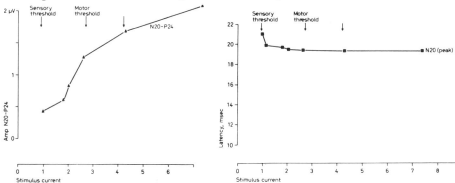

Fig. 6-12. Relationship of amplitude (*left*) and latency (*right*) of evoked potential components to stimulus intensity when stimulating the median nerve at the wrist and recording the evoked cortical response. The response being analyzed was the negative peak recorded from the cortex approximately 20 ms after maximal stimulation of the median nerve. (Reproduced by permission from Small GD, Beauchamp M, Matthews WB: Subcortical somatosensory evoked potentials in normal man and in patients with central nervous system lesions. In: Progress in Clinical Neurophysiology, vol 7, ed. Desmedt JE. Basel, S. Karger, AG, 1980, p. 190–209.)

Rate of Stimulation

A procedure in which the evoking stimulus must be repeated several hundred times to increase the signal-to-noise ratio may influence the examiner to shorten the interval between stimuli as much as possible to reduce the time needed to carry out each test. More than 4 min are required to collect 256 responses when the stimulus is applied once per second (1 Hz). The same number of responses can be collected in approximately 26 s when stimulating 10 times per second (10 Hz), but would take nearly 43 min at one stimulus every 10 s (0.1 Hz). The decision about what rate of stimulation to use should be based on knowledge of the refractory period of the structures comprising the neural circuit of interest. Variations in stimulus rate between .1 and 10/s produce only minor alterations in the shape of the spinal evoked potentials but sometimes produce marked changes in the cortical somatosensory evoked potentials.[8]

CONVENTIONS USED IN LABELING

Location of Recording Electrodes

Electrodes are commonly placed on the scalp to record the electrical activity of the brain. In clinical practice, a standard pattern, called the 10–20 electrode placement system, is generally used. This system, devised by the Committee of the International Federation of Societies of Encephalography, is so named because electrode spacing is based on intervals of 10 and 20 percent of the distance between specified points on the scalp.[9] The 10–20 EEG electrode configuration configuration is illustrated in Figure 6-13.

Designating Latencies of Evoked Responses

Different nomenclatures have been devised by various investigators to designate and describe evoked potential components. There are those who number components by their sequence, calling the first positive wave P1 and the first negative wave N1. Others prefer a nomenclature based on latencies, e.g. a positive wave with its peak at 34 ms would be designated P34. With either system a problem arises when a distinction must be made between *observational* nomenclature and *theoretical* nomenclature. Measurements obtained from a group of normal subjects may reveal a characteristic waveform that invariably appears with a peak at a particular latency, e.g. N23, and represents some essential neurophysiologic mechanism. The conflict between observational and theoretical nomenclature arises from the fact that the theoretical N23 may observationally appear as N25 or N30 because of disease or injury, or it may be entirely absent. Thus, labeling should clearly identify whether latencies are observational or theoretical components.

The Committee on Publication Criteria for Studies of Evoked Potentials (EP)

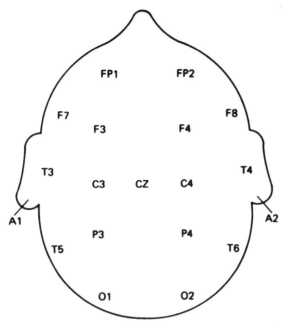

Fig. 6-13.   The nomenclature used to identify the placement of electrodes on the scalp. CZ represents the vertex of the skull. Some letters indicate the lobes of the brain: F = frontal, T = temporal, P = parietal, O = occipital. Other letters indicate the auricles (A), frontal polar locations (FP), and central (C) locations. Odd numbers indicate the left side of the head and even numbers the right side.

in Man[10] recommends that a bar symbol be used to identify all theoretical latencies, e.g. $\overline{\text{N23}}$. Vaughan[11] has suggested that an electrode label be added to the name of the observational components. Thus, a CZ:P200 component may be distinct from a P3:P200 component. The first is the positive wave with a peak at 200 ms as recorded with an exploring electrode situated over the vertex of the skull. The second is the positive wave peaking at 200 ms as recorded with an exploring electrode situated over the left parietal lobe (10–20 system). Whether the two components reflect the same neural activity is a matter for further research.

Separating Presynaptic and Postsynaptic Events

The action potential elicited either by electrical stimulation of the afferent pathways or by adequate stimulation of the sense organs connecting those ascending pathways will consist of a presynaptic and a postsynaptic component when recorded near regions of synaptic connection. The presynaptic component indicates the arrival of impulses passing along the axon and its terminals, and the postsynaptic component indicates the activities of the cell body and dendrites. The presynaptic component of the evoked potential, being the initial sign of activity, has the shortest latency, with a value contingent on the average conduction velocity of the fibers propagating the nerve impulses and the conduction distance between the point of stimulation and the exploring electrode. The presynaptic component is readily identifiable in a system composed of fibers of uniform size.

The temporal dispersion of presynaptic impulses passing along a bundle of fibers of different sizes may make the time of arrival at the point of recording vary over a wide range so that the last impulses may overlap with the postsynaptic discharge set up by activity derived from the fastest fibers. The influence of temporal dispersion in reducing the amplitude of the recorded response becomes a more important factor as the conduction distance is increased, or when the afferent impulses are initiated by stimulation of the peripheral sense organs. Under such circumstances, one cannot distinguish presynaptic from postsynaptic activity merely by the latency; only the activity of the fastest fibers of the group can be ascertained. Another factor that may seriously limit the applicability and value of latency measurements is the possible reduction of conduction velocity of impulses at nerve terminals resulting from a decrease in fiber diameter.

For a long time we have known that synaptic transmission can be blocked by stimuli delivered in quick succession. At certain rates of stimulation, the amplitude of the postsynaptic component of the evoked response decreases with each response, becoming successively smaller than the preceding one until finally the response disappears entirely. The repolarization process of the membrane that receives the presynaptic excitation apparently requires a longer time than does the membrane of the presynaptic axon. The postsynaptic membrane is not able to respond to successively arriving impulses until its excitability has recovered sufficiently. This technique has been successfully used in differentiating presynaptic from postsynaptic components of the evoked potential (c.f., Bishop and McLeod;[12] Patton and Amassian[13]).

The presynaptic response is faithfully present at a high frequency of stimulation; the refractory period is usually less than 1 or 2 ms. The blocking effect of repetitive stimulation seems to increase with an increase in the number of synapses involved in the neural circuit. For example, in the first relay station of the dorsal root fibers, i.e. the cuneate nucleus, the postsynaptic discharge of a single neuron to repetitive stimulation of peripheral sense organs (or of its nerve) can follow the rate of stimulation as high as 100/s without substantial modification of either the amplitude or latency of response. Evoked potentials of thalamic neurons, which received afferent impulses after a number of synaptic relays at lower levels of the spinal cord and brain stem, cannot follow rates of stimulation even as low as 20/s. The somatic sensory cortex is known to be unable to respond fully to peripheral stimulation at a rate higher than 7/s in animals under barbiturate anesthesia.[14]

Nerve axon is generally known to withstand adverse changes of the internal or external environment better than the cell body and dendrites. In accordance with this fact, the postsynaptic potential, which involves the activity of the cell body and dendrites, has been found to be more susceptible to the lack of oxygen than the presynaptic potential. Similarly, mechanical pressure, traumatic injury, and low temperature all depress postsynaptic functions sooner and more severely than presynaptic activity.

EVOKED POTENTIALS IN PATIENTS WITH NEUROLOGIC DISORDERS

For a laboratory method to have widespread use as a clinical tool, it must be sensitive, reliable, and provide relevant information that cannot be obtained from available safer, cheaper, and simpler methods. Only in the past few years have evoked potentials found some clinical application. A significant advantage of these techniques is that they provide a means for assessing neurologic function in the spinal cord, brain stem, and cerebrum using noninvasive procedures. Some of the more common applications of these techniques will be reviewed briefly in the following sections.

SPINAL EVOKED POTENTIALS

Electrodes are placed over spinous processes of the lumbar, thoracic, and cervical spine as illustrated in Figure 6-14 and the evoked responses are recorded

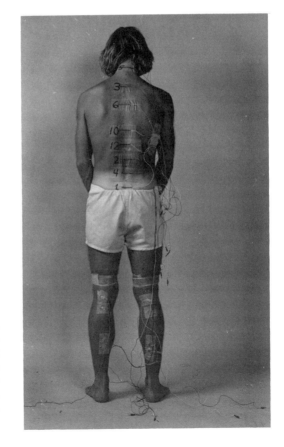

Fig. 6-14. An array of surface electrodes used to record evoked spinal cord potentials. Strips of silver, coated electrolytically with silver chloride, are taped over spinous processes of cervical, thoracic, lumbar, and sacral vertebrae. Lead discs 2 cm in diameter are positioned over the tibial nerve at the knee with the cathode proximal. Beckman floating electrodes are positioned over the soleus muscle to record the H reflex and direct motor response (M-wave) following stimulation of the tibial nerve. A strip of lead encircling each leg above the knee is connected to the common ground terminal of the preamplifiers to reduce the stimulus artifact recorded by the spinal electrodes.

following electrical stimulation of a major nerve trunk in one or both legs. Because the spinal cord substance ends at approximately the second lumbar vertebral level, placing electrodes over spinous processes of the lower lumbar or sacral vertebra results in their resting directly over the cauda equina.

With monopolar recording, the earliest component of the evoked response recorded over the coccyx is a negative deflection with an onset latency of approximately 6 to 7 ms (Fig. 6-15). This early component is measured at slightly longer latencies in the S1, L4, and L2 leads, and cannot be readily distinguished from the larger component recorded from the T12 lead.[15] The second response, also of negative polarity, seen most prominently in the L2 lead has an onset latency of 12 to 13 ms. The early and later waves appear to merge by the time they are recorded at the T12 level.

The first component is interpreted as reflecting the volley of impulses traveling over the afferent sensory nerves and dorsal roots. The large potential recorded at the T12 level has both the afferent presynaptic potentials and postsynaptic potentials resulting from excitation of nerve cell bodies in spinal cord segments underlying the exploring electrode. The second component in lumbar leads is interpreted as reflecting the efferent action potentials traveling out over

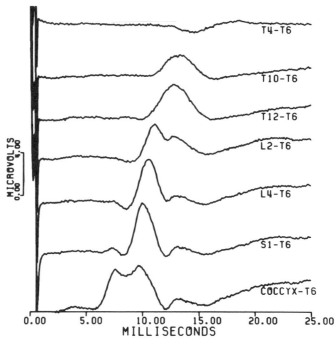

Fig. 6-15. Evoked potentials recorded from silver-silver chloride electrodes placed over the spinous processes of the coccyx, S1, L4, L2, T12, T10, and T4 of an able-bodied adult female subject. Each exploring electrode was referenced to an electrode at T6. Responses were elicited by stimulating the left tibial nerve at the knee with 0.5 ms pulses at an intensity (55 V) that produced a maximum EMG response from the triceps surae muscle. One hundred and twenty-eight responses were averaged, with a pulse being applied 400 ms after the QRS wave of the electrocardiogram to avoid interference of the EKG signal.

ventral nerve roots and returning to the muscle. From midthoracic to cervical recording locations, the response consists of a small triphasic evoked potential with poorly defined positive phases that progressively decrease in amplitude rostrally. This waveform may reflect temporal dispersion and the progressively greater distance between the recording electrodes and the spinal cord axons at upper thoracic and cervical sites.

Nerve roots and spinal evoked potentials may also be recorded following stimulation of sensory receptors in the skin of the fingers or peripheral nerves at the wrist or elbow.[16] With the exploring electrode at the supraclavicular fossa

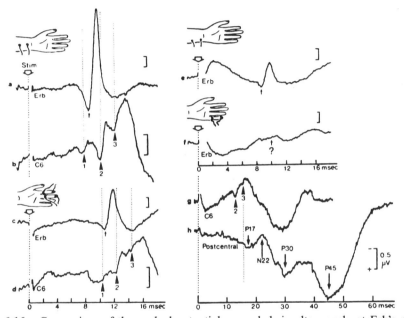

Fig. 6-16. Comparison of the evoked potentials recorded simultaneously at Erb's point (over the brachial plexus) and at the 6th cervical vertebra of a normal adult male following repetitive stimulation of the median or ulnar nerve at the wrist, or of cutaneous receptors in the fingers. In *a* and *b* the stimulus applied to the median nerve was just above threshold for a muscle twitch (0.2 ms duration; 8 mA) and 1024 responses were averaged. The response recorded from Erb's point (with a reference electrode at C6) is shown in *a* and the response recorded simultaneously at C6 (with a reference electrode on the earlobe) is shown in *b*. Delivery of the stimulus is indicated by the open arrow. Onset of the negative component at Erb's point is indicated by a small arrow. The three components of the spinal cord evoked potential are indicated by numbered arrowheads. In *c* and *d* the skin of fingers II and III was stimulated through silver ring electrodes, producing responses at Erb's point (*c*) and C6 (*d*). The responses are smaller because only afferent fibers are stimulated and the latency is longer because the impulses have farther to travel. Stimulation of the ulnar nerve at the wrist in *e* produces little or no response at Erb's point (*f*), but responses are detectable at C6 (*g*) and over the sensory cortex (*h*) when 2048 responses are averaged. Please refer to the original article for more details. (Reproduced by permission from Desmedt JE, Brunko E, Debecker J: Maturation and sleep correlates of the somatosensory evoked potential. In Desmedt, J.E. (ed.) Progress in Clinical Neurophysiology, vol 7. Basel, S. Karger, AG, 1980, pp 162–169.)

(Erb's point) and the reference electrode on the neck, a large (5 μV) triphasic potential is elicited approximately 8 or 9 ms after stimulating the median nerve at the wrist (Fig. 6-16). If the stimulus is delivered to the fingers, the Erb's point potential is much smaller, since the contribution of antidromically activated motor axons is no longer added to that of the sensory fibers. Similar stimulation of the ulnar nerve at the wrist produces a small evoked potential at Erb's point, possibly because the ulnar nerve is further from the recording electrode than the median nerve as they pass through the brachial plexus. An exploring electrode positioned over the spinous process of the 6th cervical vertebra records the arrival of the volley of nerve impulses at the spinal cord segment about 1 ms after they reach Erb's point.

Disease or injury of neurons in the conduction path causes changes in latency or waveform of the evoked responses.[17] Reduction in the number of axons transmitting impulses is reflected by a normal latency but diminished amplitude of one or more components in the evoked response. Demyelinating disease or compression of axons cause a reduction in conduction velocity, which is seen as an increased latency.

SOMATOSENSORY CORTICAL EVOKED POTENTIALS

The anatomic organization of the sensory cortex, in which the nerve impulses originating in sensory receptors throughout the surface of the body arrive on the surface of the brain, offers a convenient way of timing the arrival of these impulses at the cortex. The procedure consists of placing electrodes on the scalp over the sensory cortex and stimulating sensory receptors or a peripheral nerve on the contralateral side.

The first recorded component following median nerve stimulation is a positive potential that is widespread in its distribution over the scalp and peaks at about 15 ms (Fig. 6-17). This response is believed to be conducted over dorsal column and lemniscal pathways[19] and may arise in the thalamus and thalamocortical radiation.[20] The first negative potential peaks at about 20 ms, and is followed by other components, as illustrated in Figure 6-17. Scalp-recorded somatosensory evoked potentials may exhibit increased latency for any situation that decreases the speed of conduction of nerve impulses. The amplitude of various components may be decreased by a reduction in the number of conducting fibers or temporal dispersion of the arriving impulses. Patients with focal destructive cerebral lesions often show decreased amplitude of responses, which correlate with the severity of sensory impairment.[21]

AUDITORY EVOKED POTENTIALS

To record auditory evoked potentials, surface electrodes are placed bilaterally in the region designated C3 and C4 in the 10–20 system. Linked mastoid

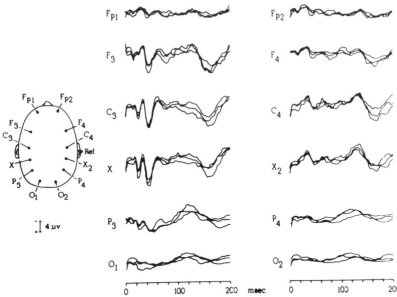

Fig. 6-17. Distribution of the scalp recorded somatosensory evoked response to right median nerve stimulation. All exploring electrodes are referenced to an electrode on the right ear lobe. The X scalp electrode lies over the somatosensory cortex. The results of three trials are superimposed. Early components are most prominent overlying somesthetic scalp regions contralateral to the side of stimulation. Later components are more generalized. (Reproduced by permission from Calmes RL, Cracco RR: Comparison of somatosensory and somatomotor evoked responses to median nerve and digital nerve stimulation. Electroencephalogr Clin Neurophysiol 31:547–562, 1971.)

electrodes are usually used as the reference electrode. The subject sits in a comfortable chair in a sound-attenuating booth and is instructed not to blink or move during a trial. Auditory stimuli are played from a tape and presented unilaterally or bilaterally through head phones. The typical auditory evoked response consists of a series of seven components.[22] Figure 6-18 shows examples of responses elicited by various intensities of sound. These potentials are sometimes referred to as "far field potentials" because they are volume conducted events recorded at considerable distances from their generated sources.

Studies in animals and man suggest that component I arises from the 8th nerve, component II from the region of the cochlear nucleus, component III from the area of the superior olive and trapezoid body, and components IV and V from the midbrain.[23] The sources of components VI and VII are unknown. Abnormalities of these potentials are judged primarily on the basis of prolonged latencies between component peaks and differences in the relative amplitudes of the different components. There is evidence that suggests the site of a lesion in the cochlear nerve or brain can be localized in many patients using this method.[24] These potentials have also been used to evaluate brainstem function in coma and brain death.[25]

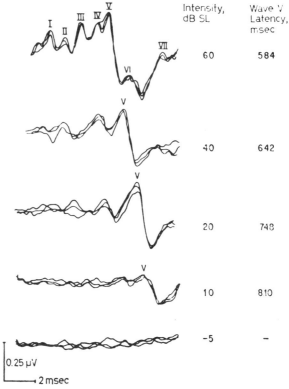

	Intensity, dB SL	Wave V Latency, msec
	60	584
	40	642
	20	748
	10	810
	-5	-

0.25 µV

2 msec

Fig. 6-18. The human brainstem auditory evoked potentials to monaural clicks (30/s) at various intensities recorded from an exploring electrode over the vertex and a reference electrode on the ear lobe. Each trace sums 2000 responses; superimposed traces are replications obtained during the same recording session. Note that wave V latency increases and its amplitude decreases as signal strength weakens. (Reproduced by permission from Galambos R, Hecox K: Clinical applications of the brain stem potentials. In: Progress in Clinical Neurophysiology, vol 2, Ed. Desmedt JE. Basel, S. Karger, AG, 1977, pp 1–9.)

VISUAL EVOKED POTENTIALS

Visual evoked potentials are recorded by presenting the subject with a brief flash of light to one or both eyes and recording from surface electrodes placed over the optic cortex. In recent years, a pattern reversal stimulation (alternating black and white checkerboard) has provided a much more sensitive stimulus than a flashing light.[26] Visual pattern-evoked potentials are now being used in many clinical laboratories to evaluate patients with optic nerve dysfunction. This method may also be used to measure refractive errors. Insertion of the proper lens yields potentials of greater amplitude than those obtained when an improper lens is inserted in glasses.

The typical pattern-evoked response to stimulation of the left eye and the right eye, recorded from a midline occipital electrode in a healthy subject and two patients who were recovering from acute attacks of optic neuritis in the right eye,

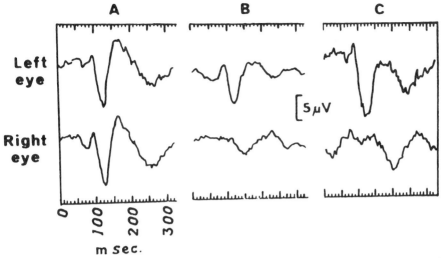

Fig. 6-19. Pattern-evoked responses to stimulation of the left eye and right eye recorded from a midline occipital electrode in a healthy subject (A) and 2 patients who were recovering from acute attacks of optic neuritis in the right eye with onset 4 weeks (B) and 3 weeks (C) previously. Relative positivity at the occipital electrode results in a downward deflection. (Reproduced by permission from Halliday AM, McDonald WI, Mushin J: Delayed visual evoked response in optic neuritis. Lancet 1:982–985, 1972.)

are shown in Figure 6-19. Note the delayed peak of the prominent positive wave from the affected eye and the smaller peak-to-peak amplitude. Response latency is primarily affected by demyelinating lesions, whereas tumors chiefly affect response amplitude and configuration.

USE OF EVOKED RESPONSES TO ESTIMATE PERIPHERAL AND CENTRAL CONDUCTION VELOCITIES

The speed with which nerve impulses are conducted over various sections of the afferent and efferent pathways varies as a result of differences in diameter of the axon, relative degree of myelinization, number of synapses crossed, and temperature of the part. Afferent conduction in the peripheral nerve can be directly estimated by recording the sensory nerve action potentials evoked by stimulating the fingers. With signal averaging techniques, the sensory action potential can be recorded from electrodes placed at the wrist, elbow, and Erb's point. A linear regression can be calculated for the afferent conduction from wrist to Erb's point (Fig. 6-20).

If the afferent volley was to be conducted at the same speed in the central pathway, extrapolation of that line up to the level of the parietal cortex should roughly correspond to the onset latency of the cortical somatosensory evoked potential. However, Desmedt and Brunko[16] have shown that this does not fit. The

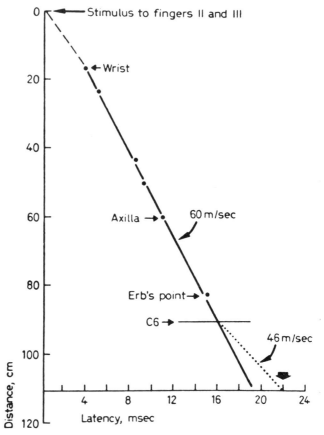

Fig. 6-20. Peripheral and mean central conduction velocities calculated from evoked potentials. Normal female subject 22 years old. Abscissa, onset latency (ms) of averaged sensory nerve action potentials along the median nerve (dots) from wrist to Erb's point, and onset latency of the cortical N22 somatosensory evoked potential component (thick arrow). Ordinate, distance (cm) along the arm, neck, and head up to the contralateral parietal scalp region, as measured from the stimulating cathodes on fingers II and III (stimulus intensity 7 mA). The calculated linear regression from wrist to Erb's point gives a peripheral sensory conduction velocity of 60 m/s. The regression line does not pass through the ordinate zero on top, because the sensory conduction velocity from fingers to wrist is significantly lower in this case. The dotted line is drawn between the time of arrival of the sensory volley at the C6 cervical level, and the onset of the cortical N22. The mean central conduction velocity is calculated after allowing for four synaptic delays of 0.3 ms. (Reproduced by permission from Desmedt JE: Somatosensory cerebral evoked potentials in man. In: Handbook of Electroencephalography and Clinical Neurophysiology, vol. 9, Amsterdam, Elsevier/North-Holland Biomedical Press, 1971, pp 55–82.)

distance from the sixth cervical cord level to the cortex is travelled at a slower speed, as indicated by the dotted line in Figure 6-20. Part of the time is spent in traversing at least four synapses: (1) at dorsal column nuclei; (2) between lemniscal axons and neurons in the ventroposterolateral nucleus in the thalamus; (3) between the thalamocortical axons and spiny stellate neurons in postcentral receiving areas; and (4) between the stellate neuron and pyramidal neurons. If a delay of 0.3 ms is assumed for each synaptic relay, a mean central conduction velocity is calculated as 46 m/sec in Figure 6-20. This corresponds well with the estimated size of external arcuate fibers of 7 to 9 μ.[27] Measurements of central conduction velocity as a function of maturation[28] and aging[29] have been reported.

Marked immaturity of the nervous system at birth is reflected in much slower conduction velocities—about 27 m/s for peripheral sensory conduction in the newborn infant as compared with 65 m/s in the adult, and 10 m/s for central conduction as compared with 50 m/s.[30]

IMPLICATIONS FOR PHYSICAL THERAPISTS

As professionals providing health care services to patients with impaired sensory motor functions, physical therapists need to keep abreast of new developments that can help to improve the prognosis of the medical problem as well as the quality of information available for use in setting goals and planning treatment. More research is needed to correlate the functional capabilities at various stages of recovery with the results of neurophysiologic testing. In addition, we need to study the relationship between neurophysiologic signs and potential to benefit from a particular therapeutic approach. Those who undertake the challenge have a responsibility to ensure that the results of their functional evaluations are valid, reliable, and retrievable. One of the characteristics of clinical research is that results are collected over a relatively long time period—often several years. Thus, procedures for evaluating patients and recording data must be standardized so that the results of each test are comparable from one occasion to another and from one subject to another. The results of such testing can therefore be used with more assurance in predictions, and the published reports of research findings become a significant addition to our body of knowledge.

SUMMARY AND CONCLUSIONS

The widespread clinical application of improved techniques for recording the short-latency evoked responses from neural structures, as a synchronized volley of nerve impulses ascend from a peripheral site of stimulation to the sensory cortex, promises to have an impact on clinical neurophysiology similar to that of computed tomography (CT) on neuroradiology. CT scanning provides a noninvasive means of looking at brain and spinal cord anatomy; mapping evoked potentials provides a noninvasive method for assessing the electrophysiologic functions of inaccessible regions of the brain and spinal cord. These new radiologic and electrophysiologic techniques are complementary—one provides signs of abnormal structure and the other information about electrophysiologic abnormalities that betray their presence and approximate location. Further developments and improvements in methodologies, in conjunction with improvements in the ability to localize generators of various components of evoked potentials recorded with surface electrodes, will contribute to earlier and more accurate diagnosis than would otherwise be possible. But, more clinical research is needed to document the functional characteristics of patients who exhibit particular patterns of evoked potentials. Such electrophysiologic–clinical correlations are absolutely essential if we are to capitalize on the full potential of these methods in the prognosis of functional outcome. Physical therapists are the professionals most readily equipped to collaborate with clinical neurophysiologists in pursuing this type of clinical study.

ACKNOWLEDGMENTS

The author is particularly grateful to Milan Dimitrijevic, MD, Arthur Sherwood, PhD, and other staff members of the Department of Clinical Neurophysiology at The Institute for Rehabilitation and Research for their guidance and assistance in the preparation of this work. Various visiting scientists, including A.J. McComas, S.J. Kopec, M.R. Larsson, C. Ertekin, E.M. Sedgwick, R. Renauff, and P.J. Delwaide, contributed significantly to the development and improvement of the techniques currently being used on a routine basis in our laboratory to assess the functioning of the central nervous system by measuring evoked potentials.

Support for this work was generously provided by the Bob and Vivian Smith Foundation, Houston, TX, the Rehabilitation Research and Training Center No. 4 (Rehabilitation Services Administration Grant 16-P-56813-6) and Rehabilitation Services Administration Grant 13-P-59275-6.

REFERENCES

1. Cromwell L, Weibel FJ, Pfieffer EA: Biomedical Instrumentation and Measurements, 2nd edn, Englewood Cliffs, NJ, Prentice-Hall, pp 63–82, 1980
2. Noble D: Applications of Hodgkin-Huxley equations to excitable tissues. Physiol Rev 46:1–50, 1966
3. Lorente de Nó R: A study of nerve physiology. In: Studies from the Rockefeller Institute of Medical Research, vol 132. New York, The Rockerfeller University Press, pp 384–477, 1947
4. Goodgold J, Eberstein A: Electrodiagnosis of Neuromuscular Diseases. Baltimore, Williams and Wilkins, p 39, 1972
5. Rosenfalck P: Intra- and extracellular potential fields of active nerve and muscle fibres. Acta Physiol Scand (Suppl) 321:1–168, 1969
6. Small DG, Beauchamp M, Matthews WB: Subcortical somatosensory evoked potentials in normal man and in patients with central nervous system lesions. In: Progress in Clinical Neurophysiology, vol 7, ed. Desmedt JE. Basel, Karger, pp 190–204, 1980

7. Matthews WB, Beauchamp M, Small DG: Cervical somatosensory evoked responses in man. Nature 52:230–232, 1974

8. Desmedt JE: Some observations on the methodology of cerebral evoked potentials in man. In: Progress in Clinical Neurophysiology, vol 1, ed. Desmedt JE. Basel, Karger, pp 12–29, 1977

9. Jasper HH: The ten-twenty electrode system of the International Federation. Electroencephalogr Clin Neurophysiol 10:371–375, 1958

10. Donchin E, Callaway E, Cooper R, et al: Publication criteria for studies of evoked potentials in man—Report of a committee. In: Progress in Clinical Neurophysiology, vol 1, ed. Desmedt JE. Basel, Karger, pp 1–11, 1977

11. Vaughan HG: The relationship of brain activity to scalp recordings of event-related potentials. In: Average Evoked Potentials, NASA SP-191, eds. Donchin E, Lindsley DB. Washington, DC, US Government Printing Office, pp 45–94, 1969

12. Bishop PD, McLeod JG: Nature of potentials associated with synaptic transmission in lateral geniculate of cat. J Neurophysiol 17:387–414, 1954

13. Patton HD, Amassian VE: Single- and multiple-unit analysis of cortical stage of pyramidal tract activation. J Neurophysiol 17:345–363, 1954

14. Forbes A, Morison BR: Cortical response to sensory stimulation under deep barbiturate narcosis. J Neurophysiol 2:112–128, 1939

15. Dimitrijevic MR, Larsson LE, Lehmkuhl D, et al: Evoked spinal cord and nerve root potentials in humans using a noninvasive recording technique. Electroencephalogr Clin Neurophysiol 45:331–340, 1978

16. Desmedt JE, Brunko E: Functional organization of far-field and cortical components of somatosensory evoked potentials in normal adults. In: Progress in Clinical Neurophysiology, vol 7, ed. Desmedt JE. Basel, Karger, pp 27–50, 1980

17. Cracco JB, Bosch VV, Cracco RQ: Cerebral and spinal somatosensory evoked potentials in children with CNS degenerative disease. Electroencephalogr Clin Neurophysiol 49:437–445, 1980

18. Calmes RL, Cracco RQ: Comparison of somatosensory and somatomotor evoked responses to median nerve and digital nerve stimulation. Elecroencephalogr Clin Neurophysiol 31:547–562, 1971

19. Halliday AM, Wakefield GS: Cerebral evoked potentials in patients with dissociated sensory loss. J Neurol Neurosurg Psychiatry 26: 211–219, 1963

20. Cracco RQ: The initial positive potential of the scalp-recorded somatosensory evoked response. Electroencephalogr Clin Neurophysiol 32:623–629, 1972

21. Williamson PD, Goff WR, Allison T: Somatosensory evoked responses in patients with unilateral cerebral lesions. Electroencephalogr Clin Neurophysiol 28:566–576, 1970

22. Jewett DL, Romans MN, Williston JS: Human auditory evoked potentials: Possible brain stem components detected on the scalp. Science 167: 1517–1518, 1970

23. Galambos R, Hecox K: Clinical applications of the brain stem auditory evoked potentials. In: Progress in Clinical Neurophysiology, vol 2, ed. Desmedt JE. Basel, Karger, pp 1–19, 1977

24. Stockard JJ, Sharbrough FW: Unique contributions of short-latency auditory and somatosensory evoked potentials to neurologic diagnosis. In: Progress in Clinical Neurophysiology, vol 7, ed. Desmedt JE. Basel, Karger, pp 231–263, 1980

25. Starr A: Auditory brain stem responses in brain death. Brain 99:543–554, 1976

26. Halliday AM, McDonald WI, Mushin J: Visual evoked response in diagnosis of multiple sclerosis. Br Med J 4:661–664, 1973

27. Halliday AM, McDonald WI, Mushin J: Delayed visual evoked response in optic neu-
    ritis. Lancet 1:982–985, 1972
28. Desmedt JE, Brunko E, Debecker J: Maturation and sleep correlates of the somato-
    sensory evoked potential. In: Progress in Clinical Neurophysiology, vol 7, ed. Desmedt
    JE. Basel, Karger, pp 146–161, 1980
29. Desmedt JE, Cheron G: Somatosensory pathway and evoked potentials in normal
    human aging. In: Progress in Clinical Neurophysiology, vol 7, ed. Desmedt JE. Basel,
    Karger, pp 162–169, 1980
30. Desmedt JE: Somatosensory cerebral evoked potentials in man. In: Handbook of
    Electroencephalography and Clinical Neurophysiology, vol 9, ed. Remond A. Am-
    sterdam, Elsevier, pp 55–82, 1971

7

Applications of Transcutaneous Electrical Nerve Stimulation in the Treatment of Patients with Musculoskeletal and Neurologic Disorders

Meryl Roth Gersh

INTRODUCTION

Transcutaneous electrical nerve stimulation (TENS) is well recognized for the management of various acute and chronic pain syndromes. The application of electrical stimulation to relieve pain dates back to 46 A.D. when Scribonius Largus described the use of the torpedo fish and electric eel to control pain.[1] In the early 19th century man-made sources of galvanic current were offered as a panacea for many maladies, including pain. However, electrical stimulation for pain relief fell into disrepute with the medical community because of poorly controlled stimulation parameters, undeveloped application procedures, and the lack of scientific evaluation of treatment results.[2]

In 1965 Drs. Ronald Melzack and Patrick Wall rekindled medical interest in electrical neuromodulation for pain control with their development of the gate control theory of pain perception.[3] This work gave credence to the idea of cutaneous stimulation for modulation of noxious afferent input. In 1967 Drs. J.T. Mortimer and C. Norman Shealy developed the dorsal column stimulator (DCS) for surgical implantation in patients with chronic intractable pain.[4] Transcutaneous electrical nerve stimulators were initially used as screening devices to determine appropriate candidates for DCS implantation. Clinicians noted that adequate pain relief was frequently achieved during the screening process, eliminating the need for surgery. TENS thus became an acceptable alternative method for pain control.

APPLICATIONS FOR ACUTE PAIN

Although most of the clinical literature reports the use of TENS for management of chronic pain, personal experiences suggest that TENS is more efficacious in modulating acute pain, particularly discomfort related to acute musculoskeletal trauma of the low back or neck, and post-herpetic neuralgia. Lampe[2] reported that TENS is most valuable in managing acute pain conditions involving the low back, cervical spine, soft tissue with concomitant muscle spasm, and joints associated with arthritis or bursitis. Gunn[5] achieved good relief of pain secondary to acute lumbosacral sprain in 86 percent of his patient sample ($N = 29$) by applying TENS bilaterally at related acupuncture points. These patients were able to return to their previous employment.

TENS has been used to reduce the pain of acute athletic injuries, including mild hip pointers, muscle sprains and ligamentous strains, and shoulder contusions.[6] It behooves the clinician to use TENS cautiously in sports medicine. Masking acute pain with TENS, thus enabling an athlete to resume play, could result in a more serious injury.

Pain secondary to post-herpetic neuralgia is particularly responsive to treatment with TENS. We have treated 14 patients with post-herpetic neuralgia pain of less than 1-year duration. Ten of these patients described 100 percent relief of pain with three to five treatments of TENS.[7] Other clinicians reported that at least 60 percent of their patients with post-herpetic neuralgia of more than 1-year duration achieved good relief with TENS.[8-12] Nathan and Wall[13] reported that only 35 percent of their patients with post-herpetic neuralgia demonstrated good relief of pain. However, most of their patients described pain of a more chronic nature and had already experienced various other interventions for pain management. Patients who have not been exposed to a variety of other pain reduction modalities usually achieve better results from TENS.[7]

Use of TENS to control pain during childbirth is a rather unique application.

Augustinsson[14] reported that, in 147 patients, 44 percent of the women experienced very good relief of labor pain, while 44 percent described moderate pain reduction in a questionnaire completed several hours after delivery. Electrodes were placed paravertebrally at T10-L1 and S2-S4. Patients with back pain responded better than did patients with perineal pain.[8, 14] Complications were not observed in either mother or infant.

TENS has been used to achieve pain control during simple dental procedures. Strassburg reported that 29 of 30 patients who underwent tooth extractions with TENS applied over the trigeminal nerve as it exists through the mandible required no additional anesthetic.[15] In a study of Brandwein,[16] electrical stimulation was applied to acupuncture points either through surface or needle electrodes. Ninety percent of the patients who experienced electroacupuncture with needle electrodes reported no pain during dental procedures, while 66 percent of the patients who underwent surface stimulation described painless cavity excavation. Although needle stimulation appears to be more effective than surface stimulation in relieving acute dental pain, surface electrodes are better accepted by certain patients, especially children. There is convincing evidence that TENS has a wide and varied applicability in the management of acute pain.

APPLICATIONS FOR CHRONIC PAIN

Confusion and frustration arise in the attempt to compare reports on TENS for chronic pain control. The etiologies and chronicity of pain varies widely even within major symptom complexes such as low back pain. The type of TENS equipment and electrodes used and the methods of application are additional sources of variability. Previous and concurrent therapies for pain control will certainly influence treatment outcomes. A most important consideration is the method of evaluation used to measure treatment results. The problem of pain assessment is highly complex. Measurement tools are frequently subjective, imprecise, prone to misinterpretation and fail to consider the psychologic background of the patient. Specific pain evaluation tools will be discussed later in this chapter.

The clinician should ask the following questions when reviewing the literature presently available on TENS and chronic pain: (1) What type of patients were studied? (2) What type of stimulator and electrodes were used? (3) Where exactly were the electrodes placed? (4) What stimulation settings (pulse width, pulse rate, intensity) were used and how were these selected? (5) How frequently and for how long were treatments administered? (6) What adjuvant therapies were required? (7) How were treatment outcomes evaluated? These queries will be considered in the following review of two selected studies on TENS for chronic pain control.

The most popular use of TENS has been for reduction of chronic low back pain.[8, 9, 11, 12, 17–20] From 25[8] to 85 percent[17] of various patient samples have reportedly experienced good to excellent relief with TENS treatment. Melzack evaluated 15 patients with low back pain and sciatica.[18] EEG disc electrodes were placed near related trigger or acupuncture points, along the peripheral nerve serving the painful region, or at distant trigger or acupuncture points. Electrical stimulation was provided by a Grass Model S8 stimulator.* Pulse rate was kept constant at 3 or 10 Hz and stimulus intensity was increased to an uncomfortable level that could be tolerated by the patient for 20 min. Treatments were usually provided one to three times per week, and outcomes were evaluated by the present pain intensity and pain rating index scales of the McGill Pain Questionnaire.[21] Fifty-five percent of the patients reported good to excellent relief of low back pain, according to responses on the present pain intensity scale. Note that Melzack[18] reported on each of the salient questions discussed previously.

Evaluation and treatment of 23 patients with post-traumatic spinal pain, 28 patients with postsurgical low back pain, and 104 patients with "mechanical" low back discomfort were reported by Ebershold et al.[17] Medtronic† and Stimtech‡ electrical stimulators were used. Sponge or carbon-impregnated silicone electrodes were placed first over a site remote to the painful area, then over a nerve trunk near the painful site, and finally on the skin over the area of maximal pain. Information on specific stimulation settings was not provided. Evaluation of treatment outcomes was obtained immediately following treatment and 2 to 6 months thereafter. Patients were asked if their pain relief was complete, partial, or nonexistent following TENS application. Short-term treatment results were not reported. On long-term followup, 85 percent of the patients with post-traumatic low back pain, 77 percent of those with postsurgical low back pain, and 65 percent of those with "mechanical" low back pain described complete or partial relief with TENS treatment. Information on specific application and evaluation procedures in this study was sparse.

In the interest of conciseness, application of TENS for other chronic pain states will be briefly discussed. The reader is encouraged to critically review these and other pertinent studies in the detailed manner previously described.

Good to excellent relief of chronic cervical pain of neurologic or osteoarthritic origin has been reported by several investigators.[8, 9, 12, 17–19] This beneficial outcome was achieved in 25[8] to 83 percent[12] of patients treated.

In addition to treatment of post-herpetic neuralgia, TENS has been used with varied success for the treatment of other painful neuropathies such as those related to diabetes, peripheral vascular disease, and alcohol abuse.[11, 12, 17, 18] Melzack,[18] Kirsch,[10] and Loeser[12] reported good relief of pain with TENS following peripheral nerve injury in 66 to 75 percent of their patients. Meyer and Fields treated eight causalgia patients with TENS applied to the related nerve trunk proximal to the injury site.[22] They reported an immediate dramatic reduction in pain, lasting 5 min to 10 h in six of the eight patients treated. Successful treatment outcomes in 10 of 24 patients suffering with causalgia were reported more recently by Bohm.[23]

Peripheral nerve injuries resulting in reflex sympathetic dystrophy appear to be particularly amenable to TENS treatment. Stilz[24] reported the case of a 6-

---

* Grass Company, Quincy, MA.
† Medtronic Corporation, Minneapolis, MN.
‡ Stimtech Corporation, Minneapolis, MN.

year-old girl who sustained a mild traction injury to the right sciatic nerve. Pain, hyperesthesia, poor circulation, edema, and trophic changes persisted below the knee for 3 months after the injury. Disuse atrophy of the gastrocnemius and soleus muscles was present. TENS was applied to the right femoral triangle and dorsum of the right foot. The patient reported marked pain reduction within 24 h of the initial treatment. Two weeks later, pain and hyperesthesia were absent, edema and cyanosis were alleviated, thermography indicated normal circulation, and the patient was able to ambulate, bearing full weight on her right leg. This author has witnessed similarly dramatic results in a 9-year-old girl with an analogous injury.

Mannheimer and colleagues[25, 26] reported excellent relief of wrist pain secondary to rheumatoid arthritis in 95 percent of their patients when high intensity TENS was applied to the dorsal and volar forearm surfaces. Pain relief was measured by objective weight-loading techniques and results correlated closely with the patients' own reports of improved pain and function. Successful treatment of osteoarthritic pain with TENS is somewhat variable and seems to depend on the sites of disease and their accessibility for TENS treatment.[9, 19]

TENS has been used with varied success in the treatment of phantom limb pain,[8–10, 12, 18, 19] headache,[8, 12, 19] and cancer pain.[9, 10, 12] In the treatment of pain related to carcinoma, the specific etiology of the pain must be defined. Is the pain radicular, eminating from the pressure of a tumor on nerve roots? Is the pain a symptom of a radiation neuropathy? The pain may then be treated with the appropriate protocol, related to the etiology rather than treated nonspecifically as diffuse cancer pain. In the future complete specific reporting of treatment and evaluation techniques related to TENS and chronic pain will no doubt improve our ability to select and successfully treat patients.

METHODS OF APPLICATION

TENS Devices

Most commercially available transcutaneous electrical nerve stimulators are designed to be portable and worn by the patient. They usually weigh several ounces and fit into a pocket or may be clipped onto a belt. They are frequently made of a high-grade durable plastic.

Units are usually single (two electrodes) or dual (four electrodes) channel models. On some units potentiometers or screws allow the clinician or patient to regulate the stimulus intensity, pulse rate, and pulse width for each channel. On other models the pulse width, and occasionally the pulse rate are preset by the manufacturer and only the stimulus intensity may be adjusted.

Stimulation Characteristics

Optimal stimulating characteristics for pain relief have not yet been established. Most commercial TENS devices maintain a constant current when connected to a complex resistive load, such as the skin. Waveforms are usually one of two configurations: a monophasic rectangular or asymmetric biphasic pulse.[27] The clinical efficacy of one type of waveform over the other has not been proved. The waveform emitted from the device undergoes distortion due to the complex resistive load of the epidermis and underlying neural membranes. Therefore one waveform may not differ significantly from another as current reaches the target axon.

A review of the neural elements that we seek to activate with TENS is pertinent. Information derived from the gate control theory of pain[3] suggests that the analgesic effect of neurostimulation may be enhanced by stimulating the large diameter afferent fibers more than the small diameter afferent fibers that modulate painful input. Study of the excitability characteristics of large and small-diameter afferents indicates that electrical stimuli or smaller pulse widths (2 to 50 μs) are more likely to activate large-diameter afferent fibers without exciting the smaller nociceptive fibers. While few commercially available TENS devices offer a pulse width lower than 35 μs, the lowest pulse width setting available on a particular unit may be selected for treatment.

Most clinicians agree that stimulus intensity should be set at a high enough level for the patient to perceive at least a distinct tingling sensation in the stimulated areas.[2, 6, 11, 12, 20] Indeed, studies by Melzack[18] and by Mannheimer and Carlsson[26] suggest that high intensity stimulation of an uncomfortable but tolerable quality effects the best pain relief. Yet, excitation of motor fibers is not desirable, as prolonged muscle stimulation results in fatigue. Howson[27] suggests that a pulse width of less than 10 μs coupled with a maximum stimulus output of 150 mA would effectively stimulate sensory fibers without facilitating motor activity. Unfortunately, commercially available devices do not have these stimulating capabilities. The smallest pulse width available on a unit should then be selected to enable delivery of a stimulus of sufficient intensity to stimulate large-diameter afferent fibers without recruiting motor fibers.

In selecting an effective stimulus frequency (pulse rate) one must consider the adaptation of the nervous system to repetitive stimulation. Fortunately this adaptation does not occur at frequencies less than 100 Hz. Higher frequencies do not appreciably enhance the effectiveness of TENS treatment. In addition, Howson[27] observed that large- and small-diameter fibers respond similarly to variations in pulse rate. To date there is no published information on the possible effects of random frequency or fixed sequence of frequency stimulation on electroanalgesia. Recent investigations indicate an enhanced electroanalgesia using frequencies of 3 to 10 Hz, coupled with high intensity stimulation.[18] Presently, however, selection of pulse rate is based largely on the subjective response of the patient.

Table 7-1 shows the stimulation characteristics of eight commercially available TENS devices. Since amplitude is probably the single, most clinically significant parameter on a stimulation device, the amplitude output range should be carefully examined. If maximum amplitude is low, the device should have a greater than average maximum pulse width to supply adequate stimulation for analgesia. The clinician should periodically verify the stimulation specifications of TENS devices as stated by the manufacturer. Stimulation characteristics may be

TABLE 7-1. Commercial stimulator specifications

Brand	Max amplitude 1K,[a] P − P[b] (mA)	Rate (Hz)	Pulse width (μsec)
A	100	25–100	35–110
B	65	12–100	50–255
C	50	13–110	50–350
D	70	17–140	20–110
E	30	50–160	9–75
F	120	10–110	150–250
G	120	10–90	150–350
H	100	4–100	300

[a] 1K = one kilo-ohm resistive load
[b] P − P = peak-to-peak amplitude measurements
Reprinted from Howson DS: Peripheral neural excitability; implications for transcutaneous electrical nerve stimulation. Phys Ther *58*: 1467–1473, 1978, with the permission of the author and the American Physical Therapy Association.

observed on an oscilloscope using an electronic resistive load similar to the one used by the manufacturer during calibration (usually 1 kohm).[28] This resistive load bears little resemblance to the skin-electrode impedance in a patient circuit but serves well for calibration.

The key consideration in selecting a TENS device is the patient's response to treatment; that is, the patient's comfort during treatment and the degree of pain relief achieved. The patient's preference for a particular unit based on size, color, cosmesis, or ease of operation should then be considered.

Presently there is no clinical basis for setting standards for the optimal output characteristics of stimulation devices. Linzer and Long[20] tabulated preferred stimulation characteristics for patients achieving good to excellent relief of pain with TENS for amplitude (25 to 65 mA), pulse width (50 to 100 μs), and pulse rate (50 Hz). At the present time, the best guide for selection of stimulation characteristics is published clinical evidence based on well-controlled studies.

Electrodes

Most TENS manufacturers supply carbon-filled silicone electrodes for use with their devices. These electrodes require application of a conductive gel and are fixed to the skin with some form of adhesive tape. The electrodes are generally adequate for most TENS treatments. However, some patients develop an allergy to the tape or gel, or complain of a pricking sensation during stimulation. In these cases karaya electrodes may be an acceptable alternative.

Karaya is a large molecular weight polysaccharide in a naturally occurring gum from a tree found in India. Mixed with hydric alcohol, it forms a solid that conforms to any surface, including the skin surface over a joint.[29] Karaya electrodes are hydrophilic and adhere to the skin when wet, eliminating the need for tape. The moisture under the electrode serves as the conductive medium. Hymes[29] reported that the incidence of skin irritation of karaya electrodes is only 1 to 2 percent as contrasted to a 10 to 20 percent incidence noted with conventional gels and carbonized silicone electrodes. He also found that the diffuse pricking sensation from electrical stimulation reported with conventional electrode systems was generally not perceived with karaya pads.

Presterilized disposable electrodes are available for use in the management of acute postoperative incisional pain. These electrodes are supplied in a variety of widths and lengths to conform to the dimensions of incisions. The conductive medium is activated by applying alcohol and the electrodes are self-sticking. They may usually be left in place for 3 to 4 days, a period of time sufficient for the management of most acute postoperative pain.

Initial Patient Evaluation

A complete evaluation of the patient's pain symptom complex is tantamount to a successful TENS treatment. The patient's medical history should include the etiology and duration of pain, previous treatments and medications taken for pain control, present medications and concomitant treatments for pain, and previous experiences with chronic pain. A previous history of narcotic addiction or current drug dependency may indicate a patient who is less likely to respond favorably to TENS. The clinician should also know if the patient is receiving financial or other compensation for his pain, if there is litigation pending from an accident that resulted in his injury, or if his employment status has changed since the onset of pain.

Next, the patient should be asked to describe his pain as specifically as possible, citing its quality, location, and temporal characteristics. Frequently, numerical or verbal scales, and pain descriptor word lists[21] assist the patient in describing the quality of pain. The patient may draw the spatial distribution of pain of the anterior and posterior outlines of a human body, indicating the areas of most intense pain. These drawings are also helpful in recording electrode placements later.

Finally, the physical examination should include appropriate objective assessments of muscle strength, range of motion, sensory discrimination, gait, function, and exercise tolerance, specifically noting those activities that accentuate or diminish the pain. The clinician can then evaluate changes in these measures during and following TENS treatment.

Electrode Placement

Optimal electrode placement sites for achieving electroanalgesia have not been well defined. Most frequently, the pair of electrodes is placed directly over the area of pain.[12, 17, 20, 30, 31] to achieve a strong tingling sensation that may be critical to pain reduction.[20] In cases of nerve root irritation the electrode pair may be placed paravertebrally over the affected spinal cord segments.[30] If nerve root irritation gives rise to pain radiating to related dermatomes, one electrode of the pair, or an additional pair can be placed over the appropriate dermatomal distribution.[17, 30] When pain is of muscular or bony origin, electrode placement over appropriate myotomes or scleratomes, which usually correspond closely to dermatomal distribution, may be helpful.[30]

Patients with pain secondary to peripheral nerve injury or peripheral neuropathy frequently respond well to stimulation over the peripheral nerve proximal to the site of pain.[12, 17, 20, 30] Since stimulation of a peripheral nerve will also result in stimulation of one or more dermatomes, the clinician must, when selecting stimulation sites, distinguish between pain from a nerve root lesion as opposed to that from a peripheral nerve injury.

Electrical stimulation of specific points, such as trigger, motor, or acupuncture points, has been reported to be effective in reducing pain.[5, 16, 18, 32] Studies indicate that many of these points are located at the same anatomic site.[33] The clinician applying electrodes to specific acupuncture points must be familiar with the systemic effects beyond electroanalgesia, which may be facilitated by stimulating these sites.

Frequently, as in cases of post-herpetic neuralgia or reflex sympathetic dystrophy, the affected region is hyperesthetic and the patient will not tolerate electrical stimulation at the painful site. Pain relief can be attained by stimulating the contralateral area corresponding to the painful region.[7, 30] Laitinen[31] reported improved pain reduction with contralateral stimulation in cases of neurologic injury resulting in sensory loss in the region of pain; for example, brachialgia, phantom limb pain, postherpetic neuralgia, and thalamic pain. Use of a dual channel device enables the clinician to stimulate several of the sites previously described simultaneously. Bilateral stimulation of painful regions or spinal cord segments is indicated in low back and cervical pain syndromes.[30] Bilateral stimulation can be extremely beneficial for unilateral pain conditions, since contralateral transmission from afferent nerves unilaterally activated by the neurostimulator takes place.[34]

Occasionally, if pain reduction is not achieved by the electrode placements heretofore described, electrodes may be placed at a site remote to the painful region. If pain relief is achieved with TENS via a systemic release of neurotransmitter that counteracts transmission of noxious impulses, then electrostimulation of any site would facilitate activation of this autogenic pain regulatory system. Electrode placement at a site remote to the pain may also be used as a control condition to evaluate placebo effects in clinical studies.[20] An understanding of neuroanatomy and a detailed evaluation of the patient's pain condition should enable the clinician to select electrode placements that are most likely to facilitate pain reduction.

Adjustment of Stimulating Parameters

Selection of equipment with appropriate pulse width, pulse rate, and intensity characteristics has been reviewed previously. Once electrodes are in place, the pulse width (if not preset) should be set at the lowest duration available. Pulse rate (frequency) may be initially set at 50 to 100 Hz, or in the midrange offered by the particular device, and can be readjusted later for patient comfort. The amplitude should then be increased until the patient describes a strong, definite tingling at the stimulation site. This sensation may be mildly uncomfortable but should be tolerable. If a peripheral nerve is stimulated, the patient may also describe the tingling in the painful area distal to the electrodes. If motor activity occurs at or distal to the stimulation site, the amplitude should be decreased until this activity disappears. If the maximum amplitude available does not yield the desired sensation, pulse width may be increased slowly to enhance the total output of the device. Once appropriate settings for amplitude and pulse width have been selected, the pulse rate should be readjusted for patient comfort. Stimulation settings for the second channel on a dual-channel device should be selected similarly. Stimulation parameters may be altered during treatment to maintain the desired stimulation levels.

If a particular TENS device offers a selection for low frequency stimulation (3 to 10 Hz), this type of treatment may also be attempted. There is some evidence that low frequency, high intensity stimulation (brief, intense TENS) may be effective in relieving some painful conditions.[18, 26] Electrode placements and stimulation settings should be recorded for each treatment.

Duration and Frequency of Treatments

Stimulation is usually given for 30 to 60 min daily, twice daily, or three to five times per week in a clinical setting.[2] A patient who responds favorably to treatment, may be taught to operate the TENS device at home. A patient should rent a device for a 30-day trial period to evaluate its longer-term effectiveness, before purchasing it. Patient and family education in operating and maintaining the device, safety, and the treatment regimen is crucial to the success of a home treatment program. The patient should be instructed to use the TENS device daily for a specified but limited time rather than "as needed" or on a 24-h basis. Twenty-four-hour stimulation is rarely indicated and, in cases of long-term use, the beneficial results reach a point of diminishing return; that is, the longer one uses TENS for pain management, the less effective the treatment seems to be.[12,17] This occurrence may be discouraged by limiting use of the device to several hours per day in a home program.

Contraindications

Complications related to the use of TENS are rarely reported. Occasionally, the patient will develop a skin irritation from the electrodes, tape, or gel. This can be alleviated by changing electrode systems, and by conscientious skin care. Despite an excellent safety reputation, TENS should not be used: for patients with demand cardiac pacemakers because the TENS current may interfere with that of the pacemaker; over the carotid sinus; in pregnancy; or in cases of undocumented progressive pathology when masking pain could lead to additional injury or prove otherwise harmful to the patient.[2]

Evaluation of Treatment Outcomes

Perhaps the most challenging problem in studying the treatment of pain disorders is that of evaluating treatment outcomes, or the quantitative assessment of the pain itself. Pain is such a personal, subjective experience that it is most diffi-cult to develop a scale to measure it. In addition, since clinicians and investigators bring their own experiences with pain into treatment and research environments, measurement scales are subject to vast interpretive variation.

The comparison of treatment outcomes from several studies in which differ-ent pain evaluation tools were used can be at best confusing, and more frequently, meaningless. However, the clinician should understand and critically view the pain measurement scales used within a particular study to fully appreciate the clinical implications of the work. The following review of more frequently used pain measurement tools is designed to familiarize the clinician with these evalua-tive measures so that the clinical ramifications of current pain management re-search can be understood and treatment outcomes evaluated more objectively.

One of the most basic pain measurement scales is the simple descriptive scale (SDS). The device uses a four or five-point scale based on the patient's verbal de-scription of the pain (nil, 1; mild, 2; moderate, 3; severe, 4; very severe, 5). The value of this scale for evaluating changes in pain intensity with treatment is lim-ited because of its lack of sensitivity in detecting small changes in pain status.[35]

The numerical rating scale (NRS) better discriminates small changes in pain (Fig. 7-1A). The patient is asked to describe his pain in terms of a number from zero to 10, zero indicating no pain and 10, excruciating pain.[35]

A similar scale, without the arbitrary divisions of 10 integers is the visual ana-log scale (VAS) illustrated in Figure 7-1B. To use this measurement tool, the pa-tient is asked to place a mark anywhere along a 10-cm line at a point that repre-sents his level of pain. The line may be oriented vertically or horizontally, as shown in the figure.[35]

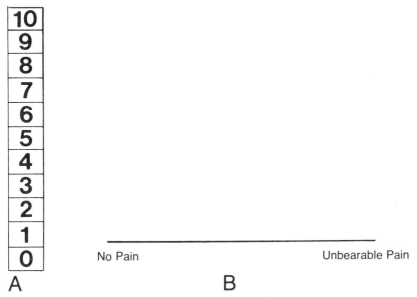

Fig. 7-1. A. Numerical rating scale. B. Visual analog scale.

Downie and colleagues[35] evaluated the degree of agreement between these scales in patients with rheumatic diseases and found a high correlation between the three scales. A clinician who wants to evaluate the consistency of a patient's report of pain could have the patient complete two or three of these scales to evaluate his pain intensity before and after treatment. Another advantage of these simple pain evaluation devices is that they are easily understood by patients with unsophisticated verbal abilities. This situation is not the case with the semantic differentiation (pain descriptor) scales. Finally, if a clinician must select just one evaluative tool, the NRS is recommended as a good compromise. The SDS offers few choices to the patient to help him describe his pain, and the great freedom of the VAS can be confusing to both patient and evaluator.[35]

Semantic differentiation scales are comprised of lists of words commonly used to describe pain.[21, 36] Melzack and Torgenson[37] developed a tool that aids in the specification of the qualities of pain.[37] They asked subjects to classify 102 pain descriptors taken from the clinical literature relating to pain into three major classes: (1) words that describe the sensory qualities of pain in terms of temporal, spatial, pressure, thermal, and other properties; (2) words that describe the affective experience of pain in terms of fear and tension, and (3) evaluative words that describe the overall intensity of the pain experience. Words that were qualitatively similar were grouped together and then rank-ordered by physicians, students, and patients in terms of intensity from one to five, based on a simple descriptive scale representing mild to excruciating pain. Although the patients tended to assign the intensity of the words a higher numerical value than the physicians, the rank order of the words in terms of increasing intensity was identical for both groups of subjects.

This procedure led to the development of the pain descriptor word list in the McGill Pain Questionnaire[21] (Fig. 7-2). Several numerical indices of the quality and intensity of pain can be derived from this scale. Since the patient is to select only one word from each of 20 possible groups to describe his pain, the number of words-chosen score (NWC) from zero to 20 is calculated. Since the first word in each group is assigned a value of 1, the second word, 2, and so on, the pain rating index (PRI) can be calculated. This rating is the sum of the intensity rank values assigned to each word selected and may be calculated for a given category of words (sensory, affective, evaluative) or for all of the categories together.

Additional information recorded on the McGill Pain Questionnaire includes a medical history; the spatial distribution of the pain drawn by the patient on outlines of the body; a description of the temporal characteristics of pain and how it may vary with time, activity, or mental status; and the present pain intensity measured on a simple descriptive scale. Each type of data represents a quantifiable index of the patient's pain experience and may be used to indicate changes in that experience with therapeutic interventions. The major drawback of a semantic differentiation scale is that the patient's verbal ability must be fairly sophisticated, and he or she must have a good deal of patience to understand and complete the evaluation without assistance. The semantic differentiation scale developed by Melzack may be of little value when working with patients who are poorly edu-

What Does Your Pain Feel Like?

Some of the words I will read to you describe your *present* pain. Tell me which words best describe it. Leave out any word-group that is not suitable. Use only a single word in each appropriate group—the one that applies *best*.

1	2	3	4
1 Flickering	1 Jumping	1 Pricking	1 Sharp
2 Quivering	2 Flashing	2 Boring	2 Cutting
3 Pulsing	3 Shooting	3 Drilling	3 Lacerating
4 Throbbing		4 Stabbing	
5 Beating		5 Lancinating	
6 Pounding			

5	6	7	8
1 Pinching	1 Tugging	1 Hot	1 Tingling
2 Pressing	2 Pulling	2 Burning	2 Itchy
3 Gnawing	3 Wrenching	3 Scalding	3 Smarting
4 Cramping		4 Searing	4 Stinging
5 Crushing			

9	10	11	12
1 Dull	1 Tender	1 Tiring	1 Sickening
2 Sore	2 Taut	2 Exhausting	2 Suffocating
3 Hurting	3 Rasping		
4 Aching	4 Splitting		
5 Heavy			

13	14	15	16
1 Fearful	1 Punishing	1 Wretched	1 Annoying
2 Frightful	2 Gruelling	2 Blinding	2 Troublesome
3 Terrifying	3 Cruel		3 Miserable
	4 Vicious		4 Intense
	5 Killing		5 Unbearable

17	18	19	20
1 Spreading	1 Tight	1 Cool	1 Nagging
2 Radiating	2 Numb	2 Cold	2 Nauseating
3 Penetrating	3 Drawing	3 Freezing	3 Agonizing
4 Piercing	4 Squeezing		4 Dreadful
	5 Tearing		5 Torturing

Fig. 7-2.   The McGill Pain Questionnaire: What does your pain feel like? (Reprinted from Melzack R: The McGill Pain Questionnaire: Major properties and scoring methods. Pain, 1:277–299, 1975, with the permission of the author and Elsevier/North Holland Publishers).

cated, elderly, confused, or fatigued by medication, or who are generally impatient.

Occasionally, analgesic effects are evaluated by inducing thermal[38] or ischemic[39, 40] pain in healthy subjects or patients. Experimental pain is induced by a dolorimeter, a localized radiant heat source,[37] or a tourniquet on the arm or leg.[38] Maximum pain tolerance is noted before and after the administration of an analgesic medication or procedure, and changes in maximum pain tolerance are noted. The effectiveness of electroanalgesia has been evaluated in healthy subjects in this manner.[38, 39]

These sensory discriminatory measures can also be used to evaluate clinical pain. In this case thermal or ischemic pain is induced in a patient, and the patient is asked to indicate when the intensity of the experimental pain matches that of his clinical pain.[39, 40] The effect of treatment may be similarly evaluated by measuring pain levels before and after analgesic intervention.

While providing objective data, this method of pain assessment is of limited value in a clinical environment. The equipment for inducing and measuring experimental pain is frequently expensive and elaborate. The procedure may be complicated, time-consuming, and not amenable to a clinical setting. Patients often have difficulty relating the intensity of their clinical pain (an ongoing, relentless, diffuse, anxious, functionally limiting experience) to the intensity of a brief, self-limiting, well-localized, discomfort over which they have complete control. Although Sternbach[39, 40] reported good reliability between the patient's subjective clinical pain estimates and the outcomes of the tourniquet pain test, the limitations of sensory discriminatory evaluations must be recognized.

Frequently, chronic pain requires more than a simple assessment and treatment of the sensory component or somatic complaint. Patients who experience prolonged intractable pain often demonstrate behavioral changes such as increased verbalization about pain, diminished functional abilities, depression, and changes in lifestyle.[41] The multiple problems of the patient with chronic pain should be evaluated objectively and treated by appropriate health professionals.[42]

Personality profiles, such as the Minnesota Multiphasic Personality Inventory (MMPI)[43] have been used to evaluate tendencies toward psychologic disorders in patients with chronic pain. McCreary and colleagues reported that patients with chronic low back pain but without physical findings tended to score higher on several sales of the MMPI, including the hypochondriasis, hysteria, impulsivity, and confusion scales than do patients with pain and physical findings (organic pain).[44] However, these personality profiles have been developed and standardized on normal subjects and psychiatric patients, both of whom are significantly different from the patient with chronic pain. The development of sophisticated objective evaluation tools for patients with chronic pain will enhance the clinician's ability to effectively treat the multiple problems of these patients.

Overt behavioral changes in a patient can also indicate alterations in the pain state. The clinician should note changes in physical measurements (strength, range of motion, gait), functional ability, medication intake, employment, and pain behavior (verbalization of pain, facial expression, and so on) as manifestations of the patient's response to treatment.

To evaluate changes in pain level associated with TENS treatment, the patient should complete appropriate pain measurement scales immediately before and following treatment. The percent change in pain intensity can then be calculated as the difference between the pre- and post-treatment scores, divided by the pretreatment score, and multiplied by 100. The analgesic effect of TENS may have an induction time of several hours, and the carryover of analgesia may last as long as 24 to 48 h. For this reason, the evaluation of pain levels 3 to 24 h after a TENS treatment has been completed is also recommended. Finally, since the value of electroanalgesia over time is questionable, long-term followup of patients treated with TENS for several months or years should be undertaken. This followup evaluation may take the form of a telephone or mail questionnaire, or of a personal interview and complete reevaluation.

Treatment outcomes should be examined in terms of patient characteristics that may effect a patient's perception of his pain and response to treatment. Some of these characteristics are age, sex, chronicity of pain, previous and concurrent pain treatments and medications, and narcotic or alcohol abuse. Careful, consistent evaluation of pain conditions will enhance our ability to select appropriate candidates for TENS treatment and facilitate successful treatment outcomes.

The Placebo Response

As in efficacious evaluation of all pain intervention methods, the placebo response to TENS should be critically examined. The placebo response is defined as the reaction of a patient to an inactive agent or intervention that may be accounted for by the factors of expectation and hope inherent in the treatment process.[45] Patients receiving TENS may be particularly primed to demonstrate a placebo response because of the seemingly elaborate nature of the TENS procedure and the patient-clinician rapport that may develop.

The placebo response is usually evaluated in a double-blind trial in which neither the patient nor the clinician knows whether the patient is receiving genuine therapy or an inactive intervention. While evaluation of drug interventions is particularly amenable to this type of study, evaluation of TENS is not. Since the patient usually feels a tingling sensation as a result of electrostimulation, and since this sensation is used as a guideline to set stimulus intensity, the patient and clinician will usually be able to distinguish between the genuine active TENS device and the placebo stimulator yielding no electrical output. This negates the double-blind design.

Thornsteinsson and coworkers[46] attempted to evaluate the placebo response to TENS treatment using the double-blind design. In this study patients were told that they may or may not feel a tingling numbness and to disregard the sensation and concentrate only on changes in pain level. Placebo analgesic effects occurred in 32 percent of trials, as compared with a 48-percent analgesic response to genuine electrostimulation. This placebo response is similar to the placebo effect noted in double-blind studies in which analgesic medications are tested. Regardless of whether the clinician is able to formally evaluate the placebo response in patients, this factor should still be considered when evaluating the effect of TENS on pain.

NEUROPHYSIOLOGIC MODES OF ACTION

Presently there is little information available to explain how the effects of TENS change pain perception. To examine the information reported on pain

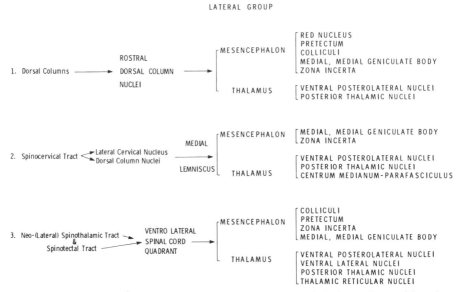

Fig. 7-3. Lateral group of ascending pathways conveying pain information and locations known to receive this input (Reprinted from Wolf SL: Perspectives on central nervous system responsiveness to transcutaneous electrical nerve stimulation. Reprinted from Physical Therapy (58:1443–1449, 1978) with the permission of the author and the American Physical Therapy Association).

perception, the clinician should first review the anatomic organization of neural pathways involved in the pain experience.

Afferent pathways are organized into lateral and medial groups.[47] The lateral group, comprised of the dorsal columns, spinocervical tract, neospinothalamic tract, and spinotectal tract, is characterized by cell bodies dorsally located within the spinal gray matter (Fig. 7-3). These neurons respond to painful mechanical or thermal stimuli or to electrical stimulation of the A-delta and C fibers. The ascending neural pathways transmit efferent information rapidly across few synapses and through lateral thalamic nuclei to the highest cortical levels along the neuroaxis.

The medial group is made up of the paleospinothalamic tract, the spinoreticular system, and diffuse propriospinal systems (Fig. 7-4). Its cell bodies lie within the ventral gray matter of the spinal cord. Conduction velocity of afferent impulses is slower for the multisynaptic medial pathways than for the lateral group. The medial group terminates at various loci in the thalamus and brainstem. The pain experience is not dictated by the net facilitation or inhibition in any one pathway but by the sum of neural activity in multiple tracts. Interruption of afferent activity in one tract can alter the excitatory-inhibitory interaction within other systems.[48]

MEDIAL GROUP

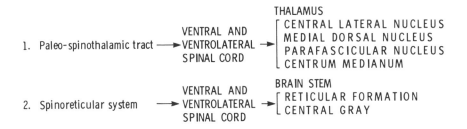

1. Paleo-spinothalamic tract ⟶ VENTRAL AND VENTROLATERAL SPINAL CORD ⟶ THALAMUS ⌈ CENTRAL LATERAL NUCLEUS / MEDIAL DORSAL NUCLEUS / PARAFASCICULAR NUCLEUS / CENTRUM MEDIANUM

2. Spinoreticular system ⟶ VENTRAL AND VENTROLATERAL SPINAL CORD ⟶ BRAIN STEM ⌈ RETICULAR FORMATION / CENTRAL GRAY

3. Diffuse propriospinal systems

Fig. 7-4. Medial group of ascending pathways conveying pain information and locations known to receive this input (Reprinted from Wolf SL: Perspectives on central nervous system responsiveness to transcutaneous electrical nerve stimulation. (Reprinted from Physical Therapy (58:1443–1449, 1978) with the permission of the author and the American Physical Therapy Association.)

The Gate Control Theory of Pain Perception

In 1965 Melzack and Wall[3] offered an explanation of how the intensity of noxious input could be reduced by a spinal gating mechanism. The gate control theory is often cited to explain the effectiveness of various clinical regimes designed to counteract pain. Indeed, the development of this theory facilitated the popularity of TENS as an alternative method for pain management.

The neural components of the gate control theory are illustrated in Figure 7-5. Nociceptive information is conveyed to the spinal cord along small diameter A-delta and C fibers. These fibers have an inhibitory influence on interneurons in the substantia gelatinosa (SG) located in laminae II and III of the spinal cord, as well as on transmission (T) cells located in lamina V of the dorsal horn. The interneurons within the SG exert an inhibitory effect on the T cells. Input from pressor or mechanoreceptors is conveyed along rapidly conducting, large myelinated A fibers. Axon collaterals from these large-diameter fibers exert an excitatory influence on the cells in the SG.

A preponderance of noxious input along the small diameter afferents inhibits the SG inhibitory interneurons, thus opening the synaptic gate and increasing the excitatory input to the T cells, augmenting their discharge. Conversely, a preponderance of non-noxious input along the large-diameter afferent fibers activates the inhibitory interneurons of the SG. These interneurons subsequently "close" the spinal gate, and further T-cell activity is inhibited. Ultimate perception of pain is thus diminished.

The T cells transmit information along one or more of the ascending pathways previously described. These cells are also under the descending influence of more centrally located thalamic and brainstem nuclei.

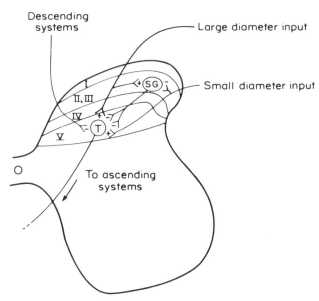

Fig. 7-5. Schematic representation of the gate control theory of pain. Roman numerals refer to laminae with the dorsal spinal gray matter. Note that interneurons in the substantia gelatinosa (SG) receive axon collaterals from peripheral sensory fibers that have a synapse with transmission (T) cells; − is an inhibitory synapse, + is a facilitatory synapse. (Reprinted from Wolf SL: Perspectives on central nervous system responsiveness to transcutaneous electrical nerve stimulation. Phys Ther 58:1443–1449, 1978, with the permission of the author and the American Physical Therapy Association.)

The gate control theory of pain has been offered as a possible explanation of how TENS relieves pain. TENS input would be transmitted along large-diameter afferents, which, in turn, would activate the inhibitory SG interneurons, thus closing the gate to the transmission of nociceptive information. However, the gate control theory has been criticized on several counts.[49] It was developed on animal models and its clinical application is limited. It also fails to explain the long-term analgesic effect of TENS, which outlasts the stimulation period. If it is accepted that nociceptive input is transmitted solely along small-diameter afferents, one would expect to find anesthesia in cases of polyneuropathy where small-diameter fibers are preferentially destroyed. This occurrence is not the case in thallium polyneuropathy, where intense pain is present in the absence of small-diameter afferents. Preferential destruction of large-diameter afferents is observed in other polyneuropathies. In these cases one would expect to find that the patient experiences intense pain, yet little pain is reported.[47] Finally, the gate control theory does not account for the peripheral blocking mechanisms proposed by other investigators.[50]

Stimulation-Produced Analgesia (SPA)

Stimulation-produced analgesia has received much attention recently. Richardson and Akil[51] stimulated thalamic sites medial to the nucleus parafascicularis in the periaqueductal gray region (PAG) and achieved good relief of chronic pain in five patients. However, undesirable side effects such as vertigo, shortness of breath, nausea, and nystagmus were observed. These researchers did find that long-term bilateral relief of pain could be achieved without yielding undesirable side effects by long-term stimulation of the periventricular gray matter (PVG) with implanted electrodes.[52]

Activation of cells in the PAG and PVG by direct electrical stimulation produces long-lasting analgesia.[53] PAG cells project to and activate cells in the nucleus gigantocellularis of the reticular formation, a region known to receive peripheral inputs conveying nondiscrete pain information. These cells, in turn, project to the spinal dorsal horn where they inhibit the T cells in laminae I and V.[47, 53] PAG cells also project via the dorsolateral funiculus to the nucleus raphe magnus within the brainstem. Output from this region exerts an inhibitory influence on T cells in the dorsal horn.[47] Transmission of information along this pathway requires a serotonin substrate. Depletion of serotonin or a lesion of the dorsilateral funiculus will abolish SPA.[54]

Morphine or other opiate agonists applied to the PAG also results in SPA.[53] Opiate receptor sites have been identified in the PAG and multiple brain loci.[55] Quite possibly endogenously produced opiates, called endorphins or enkephalins, are involved in the mechanism of SPA.[53] An increase in cerebrospinal fluid levels of endorphins has been observed following direct brain stimulation or acupuncture.[32, 56-59] Additional confirmation of the role of endorphins in SPA is offered by the observation that the analgesic effect produced by these methods is reversed by the administration of the opiate antagonist naloxone.[56, 57, 60] That TENS might activate the production or release of endorphins necessary for SPA has not yet been demonstrated.

To summarize, an endogenously mediated pain suppression system (1) is at least partially endorphin mediated; (2) involves serotonergic mechanisms; (3) depends on activation of descending efferent pathways that inhibit pain-transmitting neurons; and (4) is effectively activated by noxious stimulation.[53]

Central Pattern Generating Mechanism

Melzack[61] investigated the presence of phantom body pain in paraplegic patients, even after total transection of the spinal cord had taken place. This pain persisted after sympathectomy or bilateral sympathetic blocks were performed and, therefore, was clearly not sympathetic in origin. Melzack[61] suggested that the neurophysiologic mechanism underlying phantom body pain originated central to the level of cord transection and that perhaps the loss of afferent input below the level of the lesion facilitated the pain.

Recall that the endogenous pain suppression system requires noxious input for activation.[53] If afferent input is diminished, input to the pain inhibitory sites in the brainstem is also reduced. These neurons, which normally exert an inhibitory influence on sensory transmission, are thus less likely to be activated. Diminished afferent input coupled with neural substrates of memories of prior pain experiences may trigger abnormal discharge patterns in the neuron pools of the spinal cord and higher centers. The abnormal discharge, if unchecked, may result in unusual bursts of sensory input, interpreted by the patient as persistent pain. Melzack further suggested that intense somatic stimulation at trigger points (with TENS) could disrupt these abnormal discharge patterns and facilitate pain relief.

Other Neurophysiologic Modes of Action

Heidl and colleagues[62] suggested that a spinal reflex loop may be involved in pain relief achieved with TENS. They applied a radiant heat source to the skin overlying the left sural nerves to induce pain in 60 subjects. TENS was applied to the skin overlying the ipsilateral and contralateral sural and median nerves. The greatest degree of pain relief was achieved when the region of the ipsilateral sural nerve was stimulated. Heidl offers as evidence for a reflex loop the fact that some analgesic effect was noted when remote sites were stimulated. Admittedly, this is a rather weak confirmation of the reflex-loop theory.

Other investigators have suggested that specific brainstem loci may respond in synchrony with fixed frequencies of TENS.[63] This research indicates neurologic areas that may be involved in pain reduction but does not reveal how these neural substrates function to alleviate pain.

Finally, attention has been given to the change in peripheral blood flow in pain reduction with TENS.[12, 24, 64, 65] An increase in peripheral blood flow, noted by a rise in skin temperature and by thermography, occurs after brief periods of transcutaneous stimulation, especially if electrodes are placed over areas of high vascularity.[24, 64, 65] The relationship of changes in peripheral blood flow to an underlying neurophysiologic mechanism for TENS has not been clearly defined.

Need for Further Investigation

Effective clinical application of TENS is predicated on the clinician's understanding of current and future findings related to the afferent systems responsible for transmitting neural input from TENS.[47] Delineation of those regions of the central nervous system responsive to TENS will further enhance our understanding and clinical skill. Furthermore, justification for selecting specific electrode placements and stimulation settings for treating various medical conditions must be based on carefully controlled clinical studies, if TENS is to be accepted by the medical community at large as a viable alternative modality for pain control.

SUMMARY

The history, purpose, methods of application and evaluation, and neurophysiologic modes of action of transcutaneous electrical nerve stimulation have been briefly reviewed. The clinician who uses TENS as one modality in a comprehensive pain rehabilitation program should use the following suggestions as a guide to future clinical practice and research: (1) Critically review pertinent clinical reports on the use of TENS in specific pain conditions; (2) carefully evaluate the patient prior to initiating treatment; (3) select electrode placements and stimulating parameters based upon carefully controlled clinical studies, and your own experience; (4) record the details of application and be prepared to alter them to achieve optimal pain reduction; (5) evaluate treatment outcomes with objective measures appropriate to the comprehensive ability of your patient, and your clinical environment; and (6) review current and future theories on the neural substrates of pain perception and neuromodulation.

REFERENCES

1. Taub A, Kane K: A history of local analgesia. Pain 1:125–138, 1975
2. Lampe GN: Introduction to the use of transcutaneous electrical nerve stimulation devices. Phys Ther 58:1450–1454, 1978
3. Melzack R, Wall PD: Pain mechanisms: a new theory. Science 150:971–979, 1975
4. Shealy CN, Mortimer JT: Dorsal column electroanalgesia. J Neurosurg 32:560, 1970
5. Gunn CC, Milbrandt WE: Review of 100 patients with "low back sprain" treated by surface electrode stimulation of acupuncture points. Am J Acupuncture 3:224–232, 1975
6. Roeser WM, Weeks LW, Venus R, et al: The use of transcutaneous nerve stimulation for pain control in athletic medicine. A preliminary report. Am J Sports Med 4:210–213, 1976
7. Gersh MR, Wolf SL, Rao VR: Clinical application of transcutaneous electrical nerve stimulation for treatment of various musculoskeletal and neurological disorders. Unpublished data, 1979
8. Shealy CN: The viability of external electrical stimulation as a therapeutic modality. Med Instrum 9:211–212, 1975
9. Long DM, Hagfors N: Electrical stimulation in the nervous system: The current status of electrical stimulation of the nervous system for relief of pain. Pain 1:109–123, 1975
10. Kirsch WM, Lewis JA, Simon RH: Experiences with electrical stimulation devices for the control of chronic pain. Med Instrum 9:217–220, 1975
11. Long DM: External electrical stimulation as a treatment of chronic pain. Minn Med 57:195–198, 1974
12. Loeser JD, Black RG, Christman A: Relief of pain by transcutaneous stimulation. J Neurosurg 42:308–314, 1975
13. Nathan PW, Wall PD: Treatment of post-herpetic neuralgia by prolonged electrical stimulation. Br Med J 3:645–657, 1974
14. Augustinsson LE, Bohlin P, Bundsen P, et al: Pain relief during delivery by transcutaneous electrical nerve stimulation. Pain 4:59–65, 1977
15. Strassburg, HM, Krainick JV, Thoden U: Influence of transcutaneous nerve stimulation on acute pain. J Neurol 217:1–10, 1977
16. Brandwein A, Corcos J: Cutaneous and transcutaneous electro-acupuncture. Am J Acupuncture 4:161–164, 1976
17. Ebershold MJ, Laws ER, Stonnington HH, et al: Transcutaneous electrical stimulation for treatment of chronic pain: a preliminary report. Surg Neurol 4:96–99, 1975
18. Melzack R: Prolonged relief of pain by brief intense transcutaneous somatic stimulation. Pain 1:357–373, 1975

19. Indeck W, Printy A: Skin application of electrical impulses for relief of pain in chronic orthopedic conditions. Minn Med 58:305–308, 1975
20. Linzer M, Long DM: Transcutaneous neural stimulation for relief of pain. IEEE Tran Biomed Eng 23:341–345, 1976
21. Melzack R: The McGill Pain Questionnaire: major properties and scoring methods. Pain 1;277–299, 1975
22. Meyer GA, Fileds HL: Causalgia treated by selective large fiber stimulation of peripheral nerves. Brain 95:163–168, 1972
23. Bohm E: Transcutaneous electrical nerve stimulation in chronic pain after peripheral nerve injury. Acta Neurochir 40:277–283, 1978
24. Stilz RJ, Carron H, Sanders DB: Case history #96: reflex sympathetic dystrophy in a six year old: successful treatment by transcutaneous nerve stimulation. Anesth Analg 56:438–443, 1977
25. Mannheimer C, Lund S, Carlsson CA: The effect of transcutaneous electrical nerve stimulation on joint pain in patients with rheumatoid arthritis. Scand J Rheumato 7:13–16, 1978
26. Mannheimer C, Carlsson CA: The analgesic effect of transcutaneous electrical nerve stimulation in patients with rheumatoid arthritis: a comparative study of different pulse patterns. Pain 6:329–334, 1979
27. Howson DC: Peripheral neural excitability: Implications for transcutaneous electrical nerve stimulation. Phys Ther 58:1467–1473, 1978
28. Roth MG, Wolf SL: Monitoring stimulation parameters for clinical transcutaneous nerve stimulators. Phys Ther 58:586–587, 1978
29. Hymes AC: The use of karaya electrodes with transcutaneous electrical nerve stimulation. A preliminary report. Unpublished paper, 1978
30. Mannheimer JS: Electrode placements for transcutaneous electrical nerve stimulation. Phys Ther 58:1455–1462, 1978
31. Laitinen LV: Placement of electrodes in transcutaneous nerve stimulation. A theory of pain. Neuro-chirurgie 22:517–526, 1976
32. Fox EJ, Melzack R: Transcutaneous electrical stimulation and acupuncture: comparison of treatment for low back pain. Pain 2:141–15, 1976
33. Melzack R, Stillwell DM, Fox EJ: Trigger points and acupuncture points for pain: correlations and implications. Pain 3:3–23, 1977
34. Picaza JA, Cannon BW, Hunter SE, et al: Pain suppression by peripheral nerve stimulation: one observation with transcutaneous stimuli. Surg Neurol 4:105–114, 1975
35. Downie WW, Leatham PA, Rhind VM, et al: Studies with pain rating scales. Ann Rheum Dis 37:378–381, 1978
36. Bailey CA, Davidson PO: The language of pain: intensity. Pain 2:319–324, 1976
37. Melzack R, Torgenson WS: On the language of pain. Anesthesiology 34:50–59, 1971
38. McCreery DB, Bloedel JR: A quantitative approach to evaluating the effect of stimulating devices on the perception of noxious stimuli. Med Instrum 9:205–208, 1975
39. Sternbach RA, Deems LM, Timmermans G, et al: On the sensitivity of the tourniquet pain test. Pain 3:105–110, 1977
40. Sternbach RA, Ignelzi RJ, Deems LM, et al: Transcutaneous electrical analgesia: a follow-up analysis. Pain 2:35–41, 1976
41. Fordyce WE: Evaluating and managing chronic pain. Geriatrics 33:59–62, 1978
42. Maruta T, Swanson DW: Psychiatric consultation in the chronic pain patient. Mayo Clinic Proc 52:793–796, 1977
43. Hathaway SR, McKinley JC: Minnesota Multiphasic Personality Inventory Manual, New York, Psychological Corporation, 1951

44. McCreary C, Turner J, Dawson E: Differences between functional versus organic low back pain patients. Pain 4:73–78, 1977
45. Evans FJ: The placebo response in pain reduction. Adv Neurol 4:289–296, 1974
46. Thornsteinsson G, Stonnington HH, Stillwell GK, et al: The placebo effect of transcutaneous electrical stimulation. Pain 5:31–41, 1978
47. Wolf SL: Perspectives on central nervous system responsiveness to transcutaneous electrical nerve stimulation. Phys Ther 58:1443–1449, 1978
48. Dennis SG, Melzack R: Pain—signalling systems in the dorsal and ventral spinal cord. Pain 4:97–132, 1977
49. Nathan PW: The gate control theory of pain: A critical review. Brain 99:123–158, 1976
50. Campbell JN, Taub A: Local analgesia from percutaneous electrical stimulation. A peripheral mechanism. Arch Neurol 28:347–350, 1973
51. Richardson DE, Akil H: Pain reduction by electrical brain stimulation in man, Part I: acute administration in periaqueductal and periventricular sites. J Neurosurg 47:178–183, 1977
52. Richardson DE, Akil H: Pain reduction by electrical stimulation in man, Part II: chronic self-administration in the periventricular gray matter. J Neurosurg 47:184–194, 1977
53. Basbaum AI, Fields HL: Endogenous pain control mechanisms: review and hypothesis. Ann Neurol 4:451–462, 1978
54. Akil H, Mayer DJ: Antagonism of stimulation-produced analgesia by p-CPA, a serotonin synthesis inhibitor. Brain Res 44:692–697, 1972
55. Hong JS, Yang H-YT, Fratta W, et al: Determination of methionine enkephalin in discrete regions of the rat brain. Brain Res 34:383–386, 1977
56. Adams JE: Nalaxone reversal of analgesia produced by brain stimulation in the human. Pain 2:161–166, 1976
57. Mayer DJ, Price DD, Rafii A: Antagonism of acupuncture analgesia by the narcotic anatagonist naloxone. Brain Res 121:36–73, 1977
58. Terenius L, Wahlstrom A: Morphine-like ligand for opiate receptors in human cerebrospinal fluid. Life Sci 16:1759–1766, 1975
59. Sjölund B, Terenius L, Eriksson M: Increased cerebrospinal fluid levels of endorphins after electro-acupuncture. Acta Physiol Scand 100:382–384, 1977
60. Hosobuchi Y, Adams JE, Linchitz R: Pain relief by electrical stimulation of the central gray matter in humans and its reversal by naloxone. Science 197:183–186, 1977
61. Melzack R, Loeser JD: Phantom body pain in paraplegics: evidence for a central "pattern generating mechanism" for pain. Pain 4:195–210, 1978
62. Heidl P, Struppler A, Gessler M: TNS-evoked long loop effects. Appl Neurophysiol 42:153–159, 1979
63. Hypothesis: an informal interpretation of how the Pain Suppressor works. Clinton, NJ, Pain Suppression Labs, Inc, 1977, pp 1–8
64. Shealy CN, Maurer D: Transcutaneous nerve stimulation for relief of pain. Surg Neurol 2:45–47, 1974
65. Owens S, Atkinson ER, Lees DE: Thermographic evidence of reduced sympathetic tone with transcutaneous nerve stimulation. Anesthesiology 50:62–65, 1979

8 Applications of Transcutaneous Electrical Nerve Stimulation for Postoperative, Cardiopulmonary, and Obstetrics Patients

A. J. Santiesteban

INTRODUCTION

The great advances in the development of narcotic surgical therapeutics have not been without serious drawbacks. The side effects accompanying the use of opioid narcotics include: respiratory depression, nausea and vomiting, alteration of mood, constipation, mental clouding, and physical dependence.[1] During the past 15 years the health care community has tried to develop alternatives to the use of narcotics for patients who experience acute or chronic pain. Among the methods developed, and one that shows great promise in relieving pain, is transcutaneous electrical nerve stimulation (TENS).

For many decades physical therapists have used surface electrical stimulation to relieve pain, reduce muscle spasms, and improved motor function. Yet no specific theory of physiology guided the use of electrical stimulation. In 1965 Melzack and Wall[2] proposed that preferential activation of peripheral, large-diameter afferent nerve fibers would selectively prevent painful stimuli from being processed to higher central nervous system structures. Armed with this theory biomedical engineers, researchers, and clinicians developed a myriad of stimulators designed to facilitate activation of large-diameter afferent nerve fibers. The primary purpose of this new instrumentation was to control pain.

The purpose of this chapter is to provide the physical therapist with a practical review of the uses of TENS in three distinct yet related areas. TENS applied to the postoperative patient, cardiopulmonary patient, and the patient in labor and delivery, will be discussed.

POSTOPERATIVE PAIN RELIEF WITH TENS

The methodology used to document the effectiveness of TENS in postoperative situations varies greatly among studies. In spite of the differences in methodology, TENS is reported to be effective in a significant percentage of surgical cases, including thoracic, abdominal, and orthopaedic operations.

VanderArk and McGrath report that 77 percent of abdominal and thoracic surgery patients experienced pain relief with the use of TENS.[3] Of the patients who experienced pain relief, 15 had complete relief and required no analgesic medications. Seventeen percent of the control patients experienced some form of pain relief from a nonworking or sham TENS unit. Similar results were obtained in a study of 50 patients following abdominal operations; significantly different results were observed for the TENS group versus the control group. The TENS group experienced good to excellent pain relief in 77 percent of the cases. Stimulators without electrical current produced good pain relief in 34 percent of the cases.[4] Both of these studies depended on subjective reports of pain by the patients.

Although pain has a strong subjective component, there are more objective means of detecting the perception of pain. Among these methods is monitoring the medication taken for pain by postoperative patients. The use of Demerol was monitored following cholecystectomies in 12 patients, 6 of whom received treatment with TENS.[5] Significant differences between the TENS and control groups were found, with the control group using three times the total amount of narcotics as the TENS group.

In a study of laminectomy patients treated postoperatively with TENS, researchers found that the intake of Demerol was generally less than in the matched control group.[6] Five patients in each of the TENS and control groups had experienced previous laminectomies. Comparison of these patients showed that the TENS group also took fewer medications. Interestingly, all patients in this study had experienced TENS as part of a preoperative pain management program.

Pike, in a study of 40 total hip replacements, reported that TENS effectively reduced the amount of Pethidine taken.[7] The 40 patients were divided into a TENS plus medication-on-demand group and a medication (control) group. Significantly, the TENS group required an average of 1.3 doses compared to the 4.3 doses required by the control group during the first 24 h.

In another study of joint replacement, Stabile and Mallory applied TENS to both total hip and total knee replacements.[8] Forty-three patients received TENS plus Dilaudid PRN while the 42-patient control group received only Dilaudid. A third group received a TENS sham plus Dilaudid PRN. The purpose of the latter group was to determine the placebo effects of TENS. Eighty-six percent of the patients in both the placebo and TENS group reported that TENS offered significant pain relief. The placebo effect reported in this study appears very high when compared to other reports on the placebo effects of TENS.[3, 4]

Harvie used TENS on 34 patients who had knee surgery, including total knee replacements, meniscectomies, synovectomies, and arthrotomies.[9] The author reported a decrease in the use of narcotics from 75 to 100 percent over expected medication use. The hospital length of stay was reduced from an average of 3.9 days prior to the use of TENS to 2.5 days in the TENS treated group.

The application of TENS in podiatric surgery was examined by Alm, Gold, and Weil.[10] TENS, a TENS sham, and a control group were compared. Medications were administered on a PRN basis. Seventy-five to 100 percent pain relief was reported by 74 percent of the TENS group. A placebo effect was present with 17 percent of the TENS sham patients reporting pain relief in the 75 to 100 percent category. The TENS group used less Demerol and codeine than did either the TENS sham or the control group.

A comparison of patients who received preoperative medications with those who received no preoperative medications was made by Solomon, Viernstein, and Long.[1] The authors showed that drug-experienced patients did not receive as much pain relief from TENS as did patients who had not received preoperative medications. When the control group and TENS group were compared without regard to preoperative medications, the differences in the amount of medication taken were not as striking. These results suggest that preoperative medications should be kept to a minimum if the effectiveness of TENS is to be maximized.

Postoperative Systemic Effects

Various systemic effects have been claimed when TENS has been applied to postoperative patients. Among these claims is that TENS will reduce the incidence of paralytic ileus, atelectasis, nausea, and vomiting. The effects of TENS on paralytic ileus and atelectasis were examined for 213 patients.[11] The authors report that postoperative atelectasis was reduced. In abdominal surgeries 6 percent of the TENS group ($N=6$) developed atelectasis compared to 30 percent of the control group ($N=30$). Thoracotomy patients treated with TENS had a 10 percent incidence of atelectasis ($N=13$) and the control had a 33 percent occurrence ($N=59$). Twenty-five patients in the control group, who had undergone abdominal surgery, experienced a paralytic ileus, while none in the TENS group had a similar affliction.

Other authors have failed to support these findings. Cooperman and colleagues and VanderArk and McGrath in separate studies concluded that differences in the incidence of paralytic ileus and atelectasis in TENS and control patients were not significant.[3, 4]

Nausea and vomiting has been reported to be less frequent in patients using postoperative TENS. Pike attributed the higher incidence of nausea and vomiting to the effects of the narcotic Pethidine.[7] This conclusion is based on the observation that the TENS group used less Pethidine than did the controls. The drug had to be withdrawn from two control patients who developed severe nausea and vomiting.

VanderArk and McGrath reported that compared to the control group TENS patients were able to breathe more deeply and cough without significant pain.[3] No attempt was made to gather objective data on these observations. The authors did not report whether patients who had had abdominal or thoracic surgery appeared to benefit most from the TENS application.

Improvement in range of motion and ease of postoperative ambulation have been attributed to TENS. Active straight-leg raising on the first postoperative day after knee surgery was reported by Harvie in patients using TENS.[9] The author also reported that patients who had total knee replacements were able to gain 80° to 90° of motion immediately after the dressing was removed on the fifth or sixth day following operation. Ambulation without pain following abdominal or thoracic operations has also been observed.[3]

USE OF TENS FOR OBSTETRIC PATIENTS

A recent development has been the use of TENS for the pain of labor and delivery. In a study of 147 parturients (90 primiparas, 57 multiparas) TENS was applied to the back parallel to T10 and L1 and to S2 and S4.[12] Back pain during the first stage of labor seemed to respond well to stimulation. As the first stage progressed, pain was often experienced suprapubically. Stimulation at S2 to S4 was sufficient to control this pain. Sacral stimulation at high intensity was required during the second stage of labor but additional pain control methods were often needed. Pudendal nerve blocks were used in 98 patients while four patients received epidural blocks. No serious side effects occurred in mothers or infants as a result of TENS stimulation.

Robson, in a study of 39 parturients, found that TENS was of great benefit to 20 percent and of some benefit to 82 percent of the patients.[13] The greatest pain relief was experienced during the first stage of labor. The stimulation was of little benefit during the second stage of labor. The author suggested that TENS is no substitute for epidural anesthesia, but that this latter method is not always available. TENS, on the other hand, is relatively simple to use and appears to be a useful addition for the management of pain in the labor room.

Results similar to the two previous studies were reported by Stewart.[14] A significant percentage of parturients experienced some pain relief with TENS but stimulation was of little value during the second stage of labor.

A general criticism that deserves to be lodged against each of these studies is the less than optimal combinations of electrode placement, types of electrodes, and selected stimulation settings. Electrodes were placed bilaterally, parallel to the spine in the low thoracic and sacral regions. Although some pain relief was achieved with this electrode configuration, there may be better points of application (see below).

USE OF TENS IN PATIENTS WITH CARDIOPULMONARY PROBLEMS

Few studies have examined the effects of TENS on cardiac, vascular, or pulmonary conditions. The paucity of studies may indicate that clinicians are not using TENS for cardiopulmonary patients. Some reticence to use TENS with cardiac patients may be due to the clinician's concern with the inadvertent production of dysrhythmias. Yet, there is no evidence that TENS will produce deleterious effects in conditions such as angina pectoris.

There has also been concern that TENS is contraindicated in patients with pacemakers. Synchronous pacemakers, which are ventricular inhibited, ventricular triggered, or atrial synchronous, react adversely to TENS stimulation especially at low frequency (1 to 6 Hz).[15] Fixed rate or asynchronous pacemakers are unaffected by TENS.

Roberts reported the results of TENS applied to patients with thrombophlebitis.[16] Outpatient treatments for 30 to 60 min were sufficient to give pain relief to 90 percent of 39 patients. Treatment was given either unilaterally or bilaterally at different lower extremity levels, depending on the site of occlusion. After TENS treatment, several patients experienced return of pain when ambulation habits were resumed. The author concluded that TENS was a noninvasive and simple method of pain control.

Increased peripheral skin temperature after TENS applications has been reported by a number of investigators. Abram, Asiddao, and Reynolds noted that patients with chronic pain experienced pain relief from TENS and also experienced an increase in peripheral skin temperature.[17] Patients with radiculopathy, sympathetic dystrophy, myofascial pain, and diabetic neuropathies received stimulation over the painful area. Fifteen subjects experienced a reduction in pain and an average 2.5 °C temperature rise in the extremities.

A study of normal subjects stimulated by TENS showed that temperatures distal to the stimulation site increased.[18] The average temperature of the palm increased by 1.0 °C. The authors hypothesized that the increase in cutaneous temperature suggested a decrease in sympathetic tone with a concomitant increase in the volume of the vascular tree.

Chest physical therapy is an area where the use of TENS may have wide applicability. Unfortunately, there are very few reports on the use of TENS in pulmonary patients.

Stratton and Smith report that TENS, applied after thoracotomy, was instrumental in improving forced vital capacity (FCV).[19] Of 21 patients experiencing thoracotomies, 11 received TENS for 10 min. The control group received no stimulation. TENS electrodes were applied to areas of greatest pain; the patients controlled the intensity and rate settings. Significant differences were found, with the experimental group having a larger FCV.

In a study of three patients who were receiving chest physical therapy, Santiesteban reported that TENS and electroacupuncture in combination were effective in modifying a number of signs and symptoms.[20] Each patient was stimulated with an electroacupuncture unit during the first treatment. The electrodes of a high frequency dual channel TENS unit were then applied to four chest points. Treatment with the TENS consisted of 2-h stimulation twice daily. In addition, breathing exercises, with or without percussion and vibration, were administered. All three patients showed improvement in the subjective measures of pain and relaxation. Forced expiratory volume was improved in the only patient measured for this variable.

STIMULATION VARIABLES

Reports of TENS research do not consistently note the stimulation variables. Of the studies reviewed herein, many failed to report the pulse rate and pulse width settings used. A number of the studies reported that the patient had full control over current intensity, pulse rate, and pulse width. This lack of consistency makes the interpretation of results very difficult. The ideal situation would be to experimentally control the various stimulation variables to allow more precise interpretation of the effects of TENS.

There is ongoing controversy concerning the relationship between the effectiveness of TENS at various combinations of pulse widths, pulse rates, and waveforms. The perception of a comfortable electrical stimulus was stressed early in the development and application of TENS; now there is the suggestion that a noxious stimulus is more effective in relieving pain and altering systemic effects. Pulse rates were initially thought to be more effective at high frequencies while pulse widths were kept low. High pulse rates and low pulse widths produce a comfortable stimulation sensation as long as the current intensity is not too high.

The theoretical basis of TENS depended on the concept of stimulation of large-diameter afferents.[2] This theory implied that gating of pain sensory afferent messages would be facilitated by non-noxious electrical impulses. Subsequent to Melzack and Wall's paper a number of manufacturers developed TENS units that used modified alternating currents and stimulation frequencies of greater than 10 Hz. Manufacturers' instructions suggested that current rate, width, and intensity settings be adjusted so that the patient barely perceived the stimulation.

Recent research has shown that effective pain relief is possible by the use of a noxious stimulus.[21] A noxious stimulus in the form of a square wave direct current administered for brief periods of time and at low frequencies significantly reduces pain.

Table 8-1 describes selected TENS units manufactured by different com-

TABLE 8-1. TENS units specification

Manufacturer	Model	Pulse rate (pulses/sec)	Pulse width (μs)	Max intensity (mA)	Wave form
Dynex	Neurostimulator	2–110	40–200	50	Modified square wave, zero net DC
MRL	PC 200	1–200	60–400	100	Square wave with polarity switch
Neuropac	Ultra II	2 or 15–125	40–250	50	Symmetric biphasic
Staodyn	4500	2–130	40–100	70	Rectangular AC Zero net DC
Stimtech	Stimpulse 6067	3–150	50–250	50	Modified rectangular wave, zero net DC

Dynex, 11578 Sorrento Valley Rd., San Diego, CA   92121.
MRL (Medical Research Laboratories), 7450 Natchez Ave., Niles, Il   60648.
Neuropac, 833 Third St., S.W., St. Paul, MN   55112.
Staodyn, 1225 Florida Ave., Longmont, CO   80501.
Stimtech, 9440 Science Center Drive, Minneapolis, MN   55424.

panies. All the units listed have at least two-channel capability; the MRL PC200 has three channels. The MRL PC200 is considered a clinical model since the unit is not a pocket-sized model but is lightweight and easily transported. The other units are portable.

Pulse rate is one of three variables that can be controlled by either the clinician or the patient. Pulse rate is defined as the number of pulses or stimuli that are produced each second by the TENS unit. Pulses per second (pps), cycles per second (cps), or hertz (Hz) define the same event.

Pulse rate or pulse frequency can be arbitrarily divided into high frequency and low frequency categories. Low frequency pulse rate is less than 8 Hz. All units in Table 8-1 have the capability of either high or low frequency stimulation. The current view held by some clinicians is that low frequency TENS has a longer pain relieving effect. At low pulse rates stimulation is perceived as a bumping or twitching sensation. High pulse rates produce the sensation of tingling.

Pulse width is defined as the length of time that the electrical stimulus is applied to the tissues. Pulse width is available in microseconds pulses for most TENS units. At a fixed pulse rate and intensity, smaller pulse widths will produce less noxious stimuli. Greater pulse widths will produce more noxious stimuli since the electrical current is received by the tissues for a longer period of time.

Current intensity or current amplitude is the amount of current available from the TENS unit. Intensity is measured in milliamperes (mA). A suitable TENS unit must have sufficient intensity so that the patient perceives the stimulation. A recent view developing among clinicians is that the intensity of the TENS unit should be set at a level that maintains a slightly uncomfortable sensation, as reported by the patient.

The type of waveform may be important in determining the effectiveness of the TENS unit. Square waves, rectangular waves, or biphasic waves are commonly used (Table 8-1). For point stimulation, as contrasted with larger surface

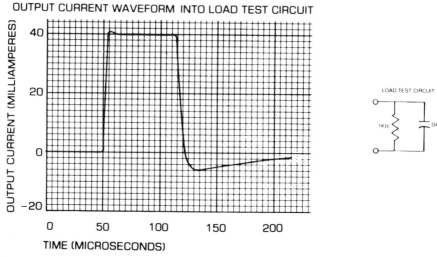

Fig. 8-1. Modified square wave with zero net direct current. Load test circuit simulates patient's electrical resistance. (Reprinted through the courtesy of Dynex®. Professional Information and Technical Specifications. LaJolla Technology, Inc.)

stimulation, a square wave direct current appears more effective for immediate pain relief. Figure 8-1 describes the waveform available with the Dynex TENS unit. The waveform has a rapid rise, square wave configuration, and a zero net direct current charge. The waveform of a TENS unit can be examined by using a load test circuit and a cathode ray oscilloscope.

The characteristics of the electrode, including size and composition, appear to influence the effectiveness of TENS. Electrodes of different materials respond differently to the movement of tissues. Carbon impregnated rubber electrodes (carbon-rubber) tend to be stiff. With repeated movement, the electrodes have a tendency to pull away from the skin. More flexible disposable electrodes adhere to the skin more effectively. Large electrodes have predominated in postoperative TENS applications. Recently, there has been a shift toward smaller electrodes for both postoperative and chronic pain. The rationale for the selection and use of smaller electrodes is that the electrical stimulation is concentrated over a small area thereby increasing the effectiveness of stimulation.

Placement of the electrodes is a prime factor in determining the effectiveness of TENS. When TENS was first used, exact dermatome placement was considered essential. Since dermatomes varied among patients, a great deal of trial and error was believed to be required to place the electrodes effectively. The patient was required to wear the electrodes with the TENS unit operating for a few hours and then return to describe the effectiveness of the unit. If pain persisted, the electrodes were shifted to another location. Alternate electrode placement coupled with variations of other stimulation settings made the use of TENS rather cumbersome. More recently, electrodes are being used over acupuncture points. This latter method appears to improve the effectiveness of TENS for many types of patient conditions.

SELECTION OF EQUIPMENT

TENS units are available in a myriad of styles, but their functions are similar. Typical units have one or two channels that allow for stimulation with two or four electrodes, respectively. With many units the clinician can adjust current intensity, pulse rate, and pulse width. Two-channel units have independent intensity controls but often only one pulse rate and one pulse width control. Pulse rate and pulse width controls adjust the channels simultaneously.

The ease and reliability with which the controls can be operated vary greatly among units. Some controls are placed in such a way that the patient with hand dysfunction has difficulty adjusting the settings. Other units have controls that inadvertently come in contact with clothing, walls, or furniture and thus the settings are altered.

Portable TENS units are powered by either disposable or rechargeable batteries. Disposable batteries are convenient because recharging is not necessary. Good disposable batteries are expensive so that the cost of battery maintenance may be a problem. Alkaline disposable batteries usually provide many hours of stimulation. Rechargeable batteries are expensive to purchase and a recharger is required. Rechargeable batteries of the nickel-cadmium variety maintain their charge for a shorter time than do the disposable variety so that batteries must be changed or recharged every 8 to 12 h. In a busy clinic a recharging schedule for many sets of batteries can become cumbersome to maintain. Nonportable TENS units, often termed clinical TENS units, are usually supplied with large rechargeable batteries. The battery life on a single charge may be as much as 50 h, and the total battery life may be in excess of 1000 h.

Some portable units have rechargeable battery packs specifically designed to fit a particular TENS unit. These battery packs are not interchangeable with other commercially available batteries, an arrangement with an inherent problem of the inaccessibility of battery packs because supplies are not located near the clinic.

The following recommendations on the type of TENS unit to purchase are based on clinical experience with many different brands. As other technology becomes available, the clinician should examine the changes with the idea of maintaining the best TENS equipment possible. TENS units should have at least two channels. The current intensity should have at least a 50-mA maximum. Pulse rate and pulse width settings should be available and low and high frequency stimulation should be possible. Intensity controls should be easily adjustable but not easily altered by contact with extraneous objects. Rechargeable nickel-cadmium batteries are a primary choice, since they probably allow the greatest versatility. Units that use this type of battery may not accept alkaline batteries, the second choice. TENS units that require special battery packs would be a third choice.

ELECTRODE SELECTION

An impressive array of electrodes is available to the clinician. Electrodes come in many sizes and shapes. Their uses are as numerous as their physical characteristics.

The carbon-rubber electrode is the most common. This type of electrode is supplied with each new TENS unit. Various shapes and sizes are available (Fig. 8-2). Carbon-rubber electrodes are reusable and extremely durable, but they are nonsterile. Once sterilized, carbon-rubber electrodes can be used in postoperative cases. Various problems arise with the carbon-rubber electrodes. These electrodes are rather stiff, and they do not accommodate well to body contours. Even with extensive taping, carbon-rubber electrodes have the tendency to work loose, or air spaces develop between the patient and the electrode. Square or rectangular electrodes tend to concentrate the electrical field near the edges, whereas round electrodes do not. This phenomenon leads to excess skin irritation in some patients.

Disposable electrodes have become more popular in the past few years. As more manufacturers entered this field, the quality and diversity of styles increased. Disposable electrodes are convenient because the stimulating surface is pregelled and an adhesive area surrounding the stimulating surface is provided. In the busy clinic a pregelled and self-adhering surface simplifies the application of the TENS electrode.

Figure 8-3 represents a disposable electrode and two types of leads. An alligator clip attached to the lead allows the clinician to use a variety of disposable electrodes with the same lead. Note that this electrode has a small stimulating surface. The advantage of a small stimulating surface is that the electrical field is

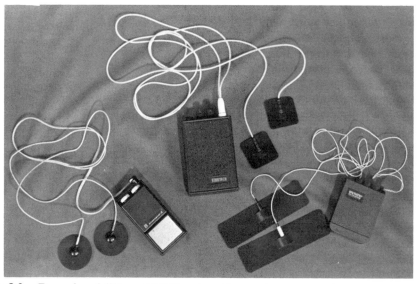

Fig. 8-2.   Examples of different TENS units with round, square, and rectangular carbon-rubber electrodes

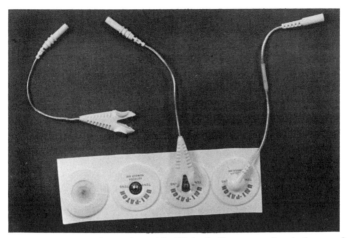

Fig. 8-3.   Disposable round electrodes with .75-inch diameter stimulating surface. Alligator and snap-on leads shown.

concentrated over a small area, thus allowing for more efficient and precise stimulation.

Disposable electrodes are more expensive than reusable electrodes, but the added expense is probably offset by their convenience. In contrast to carbon-rubber electrodes, disposable electrodes tend to adhere to the skin more effectively; air pockets do not develop as readily. Since the use of adhesive tape is reduced or eliminated, the incidence of adhesive tape irritation is less with disposable electrodes.

Many types of disposable electrodes are nonsterile. However, these electrodes and their leads can be sterilized in an autoclave at 125 °C and 15 pounds pressure for 15 min. The sterile carbon-rubber electrodes and leads can be stored, if they are placed in airtight envelopes. Nonsterile single-use disposable electrodes can be autoclaved using ethylene oxide. Shelf life is comparable to other autoclaved equipment. The clinician interested in sterilizing carbon-rubber or disposable electrodes should consult the hospital's central supply personnel.

Sterile electrodes designed specifically for postoperative application are now in common use. These electrodes are pregelled and self-adhering; electrodes are wrapped in a sealed airtight container or envelope. Figure 8-4 displays four types of sterile postoperative electrodes that can be modified for use with any TENS unit. The stimulating surfaces are large and the electrodes tend to be rectangular. This configuration has advantages when abdominal or thoracic surgeries are performed, since placement parallel to the incision is possible; however, sterile postoperative electrodes are very expensive. Carbon-rubber electrodes, disposable electrodes, and sterile postoperative electrodes should be on hand in the clinic, since they will give the clinician the needed versatility to treat many different conditions.

Electrode leads may be incompatible with the TENS unit available in the clinic. Special banana plugs and receptacles for use with incompatible electrodes

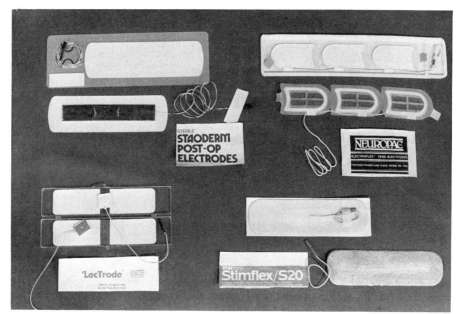

Fig. 8-4.   Examples of sterile postoperative electrodes.

may be purchased at electronic stores. A simpler method is to cut a spare electrode lead supplied with the TENS unit and splice it to a lead that accepts the electrodes to be used. The splice should be secure and well insulated so that it does not break if the patient moves or when it is handled by hospital personnel.

ELECTRODE PLACEMENT IN SURGICAL CONDITIONS

Electrode placement is an important variable in determining the successful use of TENS in postoperative, cardiopulmonary, and OB-GYN applications. In postoperative applications the site of surgery is the determining factor in the selection of the electrode placement configuration. Abdominal and thoracic surgeries are the simplest postoperative cases to treat with TENS, since the placement of electrodes is usually straight-forward. Long, sterile postoperative electrodes are placed approximately 2 cm on either side of the incision site. Since two electrodes are used, only one TENS channel is required for stimulation.

When smaller electrodes are selected for abdominal and thoracic postoperative use, one of three configurations can be used. Figure 8-5 describes one crossed and two uncrossed methods of electrode placement that require two-channel TENS units.

The crossed method may be more effective in reducing postoperative pain. Given a choice of parallel, crossed, or uncrossed placements, use the crossed

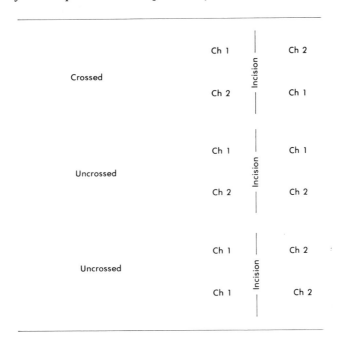

Fig. 8-5.   Crossed and uncrossed postoperative electrode placement. (Santiesteban AJ and Sanders BR: Establishing a postsurgical TENS program. Phys Ther, June: 789, 1980.)

method first. If the patient describes discomfort from the stimulation, an uncrossed method may yield less discomfort and adequate pain relief.

For peripheral surgeries and when pain relief is not achieved, acupuncture point electrode placement is usually necessary. The advantage of acupuncture points is that they appear to offer the greatest pain relief and improved systemic functions such as respiration and blood pressure. The disadvantage is that the clinician must be familiar with the appropriate acupuncture points and their exact location.

Acupuncture points, their location, and postoperative use are listed in Tables 8-2 and 8-3. Whenever possible, TENS should be applied to the same points bilaterally. With the conventional two-channel TENS, four points may be treated simultaneously. If bilateral treatment is impossible, as in cases of amputation, unilateral treatment may offer sufficient pain relief. All applications of TENS require that the patient have adequate cutaneous sensation. If adequate sensation is absent in an extremity, yet pain is present in that extremity, another stimulation site must be selected. Paralytic ileus may be treated by stimulating ST-36 and P-6.

Electrode placement for OB-GYN, including Cesarian sections, requires the use of acupuncture points for maximum effectiveness. Figure 8-6 shows the electrodes applied to the bladder meridian to relieve labor pain. The bladder meridian is used in conjunction with LI-4 and SP-6 to relieve pain through the first and second stages of labor. The bladder meridian is located bilaterally 1.5 body inches parallel to the spine, and the use of LI-4 and SP-6 enhances its effectiveness. The use of all these points may require two TENS units and eight electrodes. Labor

TABLE 8-2. Location of acupuncture points

Point	Location
LI–4	Radial aspect of midpoint of second metacarpal bone, over motor point of first dorsal interosseus muscle
T–5	2.0 body inches[a] above dorsal crease caused by wrist extension, between radius and ulna
P–6	2.0 body inches above anterior crease caused by wrist flexion, between radius and ulna
ST–36	3.0 body inches below lower border of patella and 1.0 body inches lateral to tibial ridge
ST–25	2.0 body inches lateral at the level of the umbilicus
GB–37	5.0 body inches proximal to high point of lateral malleolus, on anterior
GB–26	In supine, at level of umbilicus midpoint between tips of 11th, 12th ribs
GB–34	In fossa, anterior and inferior to fibular head
B–60	Dorsal to high point of lateral malleolus, anterior to tendocalcaneus
B–27	1.5 body inches lateral to spine on a line connecting PSIS
SP–6[b]	3.0 body inches proximal to high point of medial malleolus, just posterior to tibia
LV–3	Dorsum of foot, distal to junction of 1st and 2nd matatarsals
LV–1	Dorsum of Hallux, 2 mm from proximal lateral corner of nail

[a] Body inch is width of patient's thumb at interphalangeal joint.
[b] Contraindicated in pregnancy.

may be facilitated and uterine inertia overcome by stimulation at SP-6. If labor is not desired, SP-6 should not be used, as there is the potential for abortion. Stimulation of SP-6 during menstruation produces pain relief and an increase in menstrual flow.

TENS application following partuition should be used if excessive pain persists. The pain of episiotomy may be reduced by using spleen and stomach meridians.

Electrical interference with cardiac monitoring devices is a common problem in postoperative and OB-GYN applications of TENS. Patients who are monitored and receive TENS simultaneously present a real problem. Usually, both the TENS and the monitor cannot operate simultaneously because the electrical signal is transmitted to the monitor through the patient. This signal interferes with the effectiveness of the monitor. One option is to stimulate with the TENS for an interval of time, discontinue stimulation, monitor the heart rate and rhythm, and then restimulate for another time interval.

Fetal heart monitoring may also be disturbed by volume conduction of the TENS electrical signal. Placing the electrodes on the extremities instead of the

TABLE 8-3. Acupuncture points for postoperative cases

Surgery	Points
Upper extremity	LI-4, T-5, P-6
Lower extremity	SP-6, ST-36, GB-26, GB-37
Caesarian section	SP-6, ST-36, ST-25
Herniorrhaphy	SP-6, LV-3, LV-1, ST-25
Cholecystectomy	LI-4, SP-6, GB-34, P-6, T-5
Thoractomy	P-6
Laminectomy	B-27, B-60, ST-36

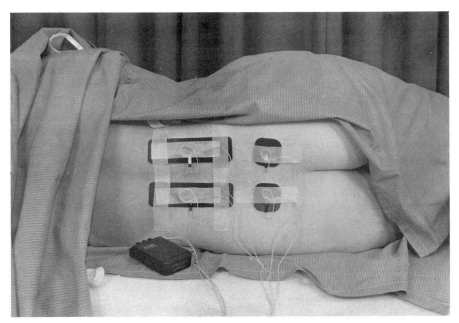

Fig. 8-6. Electrode placement for labor and delivery using the bladder meridian. Cranial direction is to the left and caudal direction is to the right.

back may reduce or eliminate the interference. Some labor rooms are equipped with ultrasound fetal heart monitors that are reported to resist electrical interference.

Pulmonary patients may respond well to treatment with TENS. Patients with asthma and emphysema, in particular, may be helped toward improved breathing by stimulation with TENS. TENS may be used in conjunction with other measures, such as breathing exercises, relaxation exercises, and upper mobility exercises. Patients who are receiving either inhalation therapy or chest physical therapy may derive benefit from TENS by the reduction of chest pain or by the increase in forced vital capacity. Table 8-4 lists some acupuncture points that can be used for pulmonary patients. The application of TENS for 1 to 2 h twice daily appears to be sufficient to improve respiratory variables.

POSTOPERATIVE APPLICATION

Application of the electrodes and activation of the TENS unit should occur as soon as possible following surgery. If the patient receives the stimulation before he or she is fully conscious, pain relief can be enhanced. The surgeon or operating room nurse should apply the electrodes prior to bandaging if crossed, uncrossed, or parallel electrode placements are to be used. The leads must be exposed for easy access. Acupuncture point placement can be conducted in the recovery room by the physical therapist.

TABLE 8-4. Acupuncture points for pulmonary conditions

Point	Location
CV–17	Anterior midline at the level of the mammae
LU–1	Lower border of 2nd rib, 2.0 body inches medial to anterior axillary line
ST–18	Between 5th and 6th rib on the mammillary line
LU–7	Anterior and medial border of radius, 1.5–2.0 body inches proximal to wrist flexion crease

When electrodes are applied in the operative field, care must be taken to prepare the skin properly. The operative field will be coated with provodone-iodine, which must be removed by washing with sterile water and sterile sponges. Adhesive tape residue must also be removed.

The electrodes must make good contact with the skin; sufficient gel is applied to allow the stimulating surface to transmit the current. If adhesive tape is used in addition to the self-adhering strip, the lead can be made more secure so that it will not pull out during movement. The lead should be wrapped in one or two tight loops over the electrode and a strip of adhesive tape should be added over the loops. Patient movement will then be less likely to detach the lead from the electrode.

Once the electrodes are in place, the TENS unit is ready to be activated. If low frequency TENS units are available, a 2- or 4-Hz pulse rate setting, a high pulse width, and an intensity that produces a visible muscular contraction can be attempted. These settings are usually acceptable to the patient, but if they are not, the intensity can be slightly reduced. For high frequency TENS, a maximum pulse rate, a minimum pulse width, an intensity that first produces a muscle contraction and then is reduced to subthreshold for muscle contraction is recommended. Evidence to substantiate or refute these suggestions is not available. Some clinicians visit the patient during the preoperative period to determine compatible control settings.

After treatment is begun in the operating or recovery room, the patient should be reevaluated within 2 h. This interval is sufficient to allow some of the effects of the anesthesia to subside. At this time the patient should be able to describe the postoperative pain and the perception of TENS stimulation. The clinician may have to readjust the intensity controls, usually upward, so that the patient is able to perceive the stimulation. The patient should not be encouraged to manipulate the controls. These settings should be controlled only by the therapist.

Stimulation may be continuous or at intervals, such as 2 h on, 2 h off. For the first day the electrodes should remain in place. If sterile long-lasting electrodes are used, they may be kept in place up to 3 days. The electrode site should be checked daily, if possible, to determine the presence of skin irritation, adequate electrode contact, and continuity of adhesive tape. Faulty electrodes should be replaced, and inadequate electrode placement rectified.

Three days of intermittent or continuous stimulation is sufficient in most postoperative cases. Additional stimulation may be required in different cases and some patients may require the use of a TENS on a home program. The patient will require indepth instruction on how to maintain and adjust the unit.

Postoperative TENS Evaluation

Patient _____   Date _____

Diagnosis_____   Surgical Procedure_____

Medication History_____

Electrode Placement:

    Immediate Post Op:_____

    Changes:_____ Date _____

Current Intensity _____ Pulse Rate _____ Pulse Width _____

Medications: PRN or scheduled

List of medications: _____

Medication Intake: Time/Dose/Type

    Day 1: _____

    Day 2: _____

    Day 3: _____

Report of Pain: Time/Severity

_____

Mobility: _____

Atelectasis: Yes _____ No _____   Ileus: Yes _____   No _____

Stimulation Terminated on_____

Fig. 8-7. Components of a patient evaluation form for postoperative TENS.

It is exceedingly important to document the effectiveness of the TENS. The type of surgery, the electrode placement, control settings, number of medications, patient responses to stimulation, breathing, and mobility are variables that must be documented. Figure 8-7 represents a suggested documentation form for TENS.

If a TENS postoperative program is being utilized, the physical therapist may wish to expand service to different types of surgeries as well as to labor and delivery. The clinician must make a significant effort so that service is rendered promptly and accurately and that documentation is maintained. Data on the effectiveness of postoperative TENS are useful in promoting the program.

Research articles and inservice presentations are two methods of informing medical colleagues about TENS. A set of research articles compiled and distributed to referring physicians will help to inform them about this modality.

SUMMARY

The literature has shown that TENS is effective for managing pain following surgery. TENS appears to be effective in labor and delivery as well. Little information is available on the effects of TENS for pulmonary and cardiac patients, but there appears to be potential for the relief of breathing dysfunction in emphysema and asthma.

A number of TENS units and different stimulation variables are reviewed. Four-channel, low frequency TENS units are recommended. Small, round electrodes may be more effective, especially when used over acupuncture points. Various electrode placements for postsurgical, labor and delivery, and pulmonary conditions are described. Acupuncture point stimulation is recommended for most conditions, but patients who have had thoracic and abdominal operations respond well to parallel, crossed, or uncrossed electrode placements.

REFERENCES

1. Solomon RA, Viernstein MC, Long DM: Reduction of postoperative pain and narcotic use by transcutaneous electrical nerve stimulation. Surgery 87: 142–145, 1980
2. Melzack R, Wall PD: Pain mechanisms: a new theory. Science 150: 971–979, 1965
3. VanderArk GD, McGrath KA: Transcutaneous electrical stimulation in treatment of postoperative pain. Am J Surg 130: 338–340, 1975
4. Cooperman AM, Hall B, Sadar, ES, et al: Use of transcutaneous electrical stimulation in control of postoperative pain. Surg Forum 26: 77–78, 1975
5. Rosenberg M, Curtis L, Bourke DL: Transcuteaneous electrical nerve stimulation for the relief of postoperative pain. Pain 5:129–133, 1978
6. Boulos MI, Leroy PL, Goloskov J, et al: Neuromodulation for the control of postoperative pain and muscle spasm. In Current Concepts in the Management of Chronic Pain, ed. LeRoy PL, Symposia Specialists, Miami, FL, 1977
7. Pike PMH: Transcutaneous electrical stimulation: Its use in the management of postoperative pain. Anaesthesia 33:165–171, 1978
8. Stabile, ML, Mallory, TH: The management of postoperative pain in total joint replacement. Orthopaedic Rev 7:121–123, 1978.
9. Harvie KW: A major advance in the control of postoperative knee pain. Orthopedics 2: 129–131, 1979
10. Alm WA, Gold ML, Weil LS: Evaluation of transcutaneous electrical nerve stimulation (TENS) in podiatric surgery: J Am Podiatry Assoc 69:537–542, 1979
11. Hymes AC, Yonehiro EG, Raab DE, et al: Electrical surface stimulation for treatment and prevention of ileus and atelectasis. Surg Forum 25: 222–224, 1974
12. Augustinsson LE, Bohlin P, Budsen P, et al: Pain relief during delivery by transcutaneous electrical nerve stimulation. Pain 4:59–65, 1977
13. Robson JE: Transcutaneous nerve stimulation for pain relief in labour. Anaesthesia 34:357–360, 1979
14. Steward P: Transcutaneous nerve stimulation as a method of analgesia in labour. Anaesthesia 34:361–364, 1979
15. Eriksson M, Schuller H, Sjölund B: Hazard from transcutaneous nerve stimulation in patients with pacemakers. Lacet 1: 1319, 1978
16. Roberts HJ: Transcutaneous electrical nerve stimulation in the symptomatic management of thrombophlebitis. Angiology 30:249–256, 1979
17. Abram SE, Adiddao CB, Reynolds AC: Increased skin temperature during transcutaneous electrical stimulation. Anesth Analg 59:1, 1980
18. Owens D, Atkinson ER, Lees DE: Thermographic evidence of reduced sympathetic tone with transcutaneous nerve stimulation. Anesthesiology 50: 62–65, 1979

19. Stratton SA, Smith MA: Effect of transcutaneous electrical nerve stimulation on forced vital capacity. Phys Ther 60: 45–47, 1980
20. Santiesteban AJ: Electroacupuncture in chest physical therapy: three case studies. Paper presented at midwinter meeting of American Physical Therapy Association, New Orleans, February, 1980.
21. Santiesteban AJ: Electroacupuncture and low back pain. Paper presented at national meeting of American Physical Therapy Association, Phoenix, AZ, June 1980

Index

Page numbers followed by f represent figures; page numbers followed by t represent tables. Page numbers in bold type represent definitions.